Talking with Doctors

David Newman

THE ANALYTIC PRESS

2006   Hillsdale, NJ   London

Published by
The Analytic Press, Inc., Publishers
    Editorial Offices:
    101 West Street
    Hillsdale, NJ 07642

    www.analyticpress.com

Designed and typeset (Garamond, Palatino) by
Christopher Jaworski, Bloomfield, NJ, qualitext@verizon.net

**Library of Congress
Cataloging-in-Publication Data**

Newman, David, 1955–
    Talking with doctors / David Newman
       p. cm.
    ISBN 0–88163–446–8
    1. Newman, David, 1955—Health. 2. Psychoanalysts—
New York (State)—New York—Biography. 3. Skull—
Tumors—Patients—New York (State)—New York—
Biography. 4. Physician and patient. I. Title.

    RC339.52.N47A3 2006
    362.196'9947150092—dc22
    [B]

                                  2005053099

Printed in the United States of America
10 9 8 7 6 5 4 3 2 1

To Jacob, Isaiah, and Judah, and to Suzie

Contents

Author's Note

*I*n the text that follows, I have changed the names of many people to protect their confidentiality and privacy. For similar reasons, I have changed minor identifying details of several individuals and places. Except for such alterations, the story has been reconstructed with as much accuracy as possible, using my records, my memory, and the memory of others who participated in my efforts at the time.

Talking with Doctors

In early September 1999 I was told I had a large, malignant, life-threatening tumor in the center of my skull. It was, when discovered, within one or two millimeters of the brain stem, which controls involuntary functions like breathing, and the carotid artery, which carries blood to the brain. Several prominent doctors said the tumor was inoperable, and they were skeptical about the potential effectiveness of chemotherapy and radiation. One well-known physician cautioned that I should get my "affairs in order," that I might have only a 10% chance of surviving two years. I was 44 at the time, married, and the father of three young children.

I sought other medical opinions. I live in New York, and in a period of five weeks I consulted at four major medical institutions. I met with a host of doctors with various specializations. These encounters lasted an hour and a half at most, sometimes one hour or less. It was a very short time in which to decide who to trust my life with, who to rely on, who could genuinely help. As one might expect, there were differences of perspective, some widely divergent, differences which often required strenuous effort to define and clarify. I was desperate, medically ignorant, and intensely vulnerable, and all the doctors I spoke with sought to be convincing and authoritative, even about their uncertainties. Their offhand remarks and incidental behaviors were charged with meanings for me—meanings that I often had difficulty deciphering but which just as frequently revealed far more than was intended.

These were intimate and intense life-and-death dialogues with strangers, doctors with whom no adequate basis for personal trust had ever been established. While I did not wish to face the nearly impossible task of assessing a physician's competence, experience, and wisdom, I had to choose in whose hands to put my life.

What follows was written from memory, with periodic reference to an appointment calendar and several torn scraps of paper. The latter contain questions written down prior to my consultations with the doctors. These notes are repetitive, lifeless, focused on risks and benefits of suggested courses of action. They describe nothing of my interaction with the physicians and contain nothing of my feelings regarding the imminence of my disappearance and abandonment of those I love.

They do, however, provide a chronological sequence that I use to structure the story. The sequence of dates gives a genuine order and progression, but one that is deceptive. I didn't know where I was going, and I didn't know how I was going to get there. Neither did I know how much time I had.

I felt my way, as one might down a dark alley, using all my senses.

Please Give Him Back His Copay

In the three months prior to the initial diagnosis, I had a few very brief spontaneous nosebleeds. One in June, two in July, each lasting less than a minute. I was previously not prone to nosebleeds and had recently been put on a cholesterol-lowering medication. Wondering if nosebleeds might be a side effect, I called my internist, had a blood test, which was negative, and was then referred to an ENT specialist who looked up my nose and, hypothesizing that there was a polyp, requested a CT scan.

One week later, on September 9th, 1999, I entered Dr. Gibson's office. He put three film sheets on the light screens and quickly announced, "You have a large tumor, five to six centimeters in diameter, in your sinus cavities and at the base of your skull. It has destroyed a lot of tissue and bone and is adjacent to the cavernous sinus, which contains the carotid artery, which carries blood to the brain. It abuts the nerves to your eyes ... sits on the optic chiasm ... and it has broken through the bone that protects your brain. Your survival is at stake."

While I tried desperately to orient myself before the images and listen very carefully to what was being said, I almost immediately felt numb—in a haze, a transparent shell. In one moment everything about my life changed. Suddenly I was made privy to a world inside my head about which I hadn't a clue. Dr. Gibson looked nervous and awkward and became increasingly so. He spoke haltingly and then appeared uncertain, not only about what, but about how, he was communicating. At first he seemed unsure about how he wished to proceed, but then, with an increasing sense of urgency, decided he should do a biopsy *"right away, on the spot."* He asserted, "If you were my brother, I would want it done *immediately!"*

The rhetorical gambit of treating me like family was one I would encounter several times in the following weeks. It was meant to convey personal regard and to inspire trust. The physician was saying he was relating to me with a profound degree of care and concern. He was implicitly conveying, "Trust me here. My motives are clear." Yet such remarks tended to be used in moments of immense tension and doubt. The sight of my confusion and uncertainty, of my giving thought to something, or even my momentary silence, appeared to precipitate a reaction in the doctor, and such assertions were made to quiet fears—including those of the physician himself.

Although I did not know, or even consider, the complications such a biopsy might involve, I hesitantly agreed to go ahead with the procedure. In other words, I was initially convinced by Dr. Gibson's rhetoric. In the preceding few moments I had been asked to look at images I could not grasp, had tried to orient myself to anatomy I had never encountered, and had struggled to assimilate the threat to my life—and I was now ready to trust a doctor I didn't know.

But Dr. Gibson himself reconsidered: "Dr. Scheuer, the most experienced physician in the department, knows more about this than I do. He should do the biopsy. Let me see if he's around." The doctor then left me and my mind alone in the consulting room. I was baffled by his apparent absence of preparation (the films and radiologist's report had been in his possession for over a week), and I was unsettled by his shift of intention. I waited trembling. Ten minutes later Dr. Gibson returned, having arranged for me to see the more senior physician the following afternoon. He told me that he had been able to get an appointment so soon with Dr. Scheuer (who ordinarily was booked weeks in advance) only because of the urgency of my case.

Gibson next asked me to follow him into his receptionist's office. He sat down at a computer, immediately began typing, and only then turned slightly toward me: "I'm sorry for being so blunt, but your life *is* at stake. The tumor is adjacent to several vital organs." Swiveling in his chair, he addressed his receptionist: "Please give him back his copay."

I accepted this stupefying non sequitur with robotlike compliance. Like an automaton, I took the 10 dollars handed to me, wondering why this mattered at the moment. It felt like an uncanny, mystifying payoff. Whether it was motivated by the doctor's guilt or generosity or pity, I still felt more than a hint of being erased.

Seeking some personal contact, and in an effort to overcome the feeling of isolation, of having been dismissed, I turned to Dr. Gibson, who was again typing at his computer. I asked if I would be seeing him again. Surprised, taken aback, he said, "Sure . . . if you want to . . . although you probably won't want to. . . . Why not wait til after tomorrow to schedule something . . . after you see Dr. Scheuer. . . ."

Like the rest of us, doctors can fail to exercise forethought, be ill-prepared, speak impulsively, and make obscure attempts at reparation. As soon as I could, I put those 10 dollars, the returned copay, into an interest-bearing account earmarked for purchase of my gravesite.

The Worst-Case Scenario

*F*ollowing the consultation with Dr. Gibson, I went, in a state of shock, to my primary-care physician's office in the same building. Even in such a circumstance, I was scrupulous in my efforts to get that essential piece of paper, a new referral. Obviously the receptionists had no inkling of my state of mind. When I left the building, I searched for a pay phone. I remember the blinding brightness of the sunlight. I called my wife, Suzie. A nursery school director, she was in her office with our oldest son, Jacob (who was nine), because it was early September and his school had not yet begun. I told her it was an emergency and she should speak in private. Shaking and crying, I described what I had heard and arranged to see her as soon as possible. When I went to the parking lot to retrieve my car, I couldn't find my ticket. Then, after paying, I couldn't find my receipt (to get out of the lot), and, trembling, walked back and forth searching the ground.

I drove to my office, which was close to Suzie's school. I am a psychotherapist and had appointments with several patients later that afternoon. When I arrived I called Suzie and walked over to her office. We spoke briefly in Jacob's absence and then, as he knew something was up, in his presence. We gave a very general description of my medical situation. He asked several questions, matter-of-factly, and then, "If it is cancer, what's the worst-case scenario?" To this, Suzie or I mumbled something like, "Well, it may very well be curable," to which Jacob responded, "And it may not?"

In the days and weeks to follow I forgot that conversation, several times. When people asked me about my children, I failed to recall Jacob's immediate, penetrating inquiry and focused on his subsequent restraint, his apparent distance, and the lack of specific, detailed questions, which were ordinarily his hallmark.

Forewarned, Four-Armed

At many points in the weeks following my departure from Dr. Gibson's office, it seemed that an invisible, unknowable, mammoth lurked in every room, on every street. The sensation was that an insurmountable barrier, blinding and confining, existed between everybody else and me. I felt as though I were partially entombed. Something appeared inherently wrong in my perceptions and experience. When with others, I often sensed I was marked for death. Whatever the overt empathy, there was an unintended distance; their lives were expected to continue.

Naturally Suzie and I sought, over the next several weeks, to be as protective as possible of our three children (Jacob, nine, and Judah and Isaiah, both three and a half).

This meant not speaking of my illness in their presence, particularly while there was tremendous uncertainty and the viability of any treatment was unclear. Doing so was difficult, as I was frequently on the phone and people visited our home.

By contrast, outside the home and the presence of our children, Suzie and I spoke with anyone we thought could be of help. Our conversations ranged from those with close friends to those with distant acquaintances or people we didn't know but were put in touch with. The worst-case scenario almost led me to abandon my customary social restraint.

Of the people who helped me through the anxiety and fear, it was Suzie who was with me the most. It was she who bore the brunt of my trembling, she who I leaned on. Suzie had her own worries and fearful imaginings, but they did not interfere with her being consistently present and caring. She kept our home stable and loving, and she accompanied me to every subsequent consultation that fall. The people at her school understood the nature of this crisis and knew that Suzie would do everything she could to make sure things ran smoothly at work, even in her absence. The staff and teachers worked together to make this happen. At a staff meeting Suzie told her assembled teachers, in response to their offers of help, "The most important thing you can do for me is to keep everything here running well." She kept close track of what was going on, but others assumed some of her responsibilities, and she was given the opportunity to be with me.

Suzie and I, in our 11 years together, had plenty of experience with medical emergencies. Having met when we were both 32 (she, a dancer, part-time teacher, and waitress; I, a painter and part-time teacher), we were eager to have a family and married less than 10 months after our first blind date and the handful of conversations that quickly established our mutual excitement in finding someone with whom we could be close. Exactly two years following that initial meeting, we brought our first child home from the hospital. In the next nine years, we had two late miscarriages, two complicated deliveries, and one very sick child. These experiences lay in the background and no doubt informed our responses to my medical emergency.

Jacob, our first child, had been delivered by emergency C-section because the umbilical cord was wrapped around his neck, and when Suzie pushed, his heart beat dropped precipitously. Suzie's next pregnancy ended in miscarriage in the fifth month. We were hurt by the coldness and impersonal manner of the covering physician (our own doctor was away on vacation), and our hearts were torn by the loss and disappointment. Our obstetrician told us that there was no way of knowing what had caused the miscarriage, although it had occurred 10 days after an amniocentesis. This obstetrician, well known for handling high-risk cases, assured us, "Don't worry. Lightning doesn't strike twice in the same place."

But it did: Suzie's next pregnancy ended in miscarriage in the fifth month. Our doctor, again away, was informed by the covering physician but failed to call and speak with us for several days. When we met with her weeks later, she asserted, whether out of legal or professional wisdom, that she would do nothing differently the next pregnancy. Her manner, which had previously been so warm and friendly, now appeared dissembling; she seemed to be acting as though nothing had happened. I recall being in her office, cluttered with pictures of her family, her usual jovial style marginally inhibited. I remember feeling she never again spoke openly with us, and we were disappointed, distrustful, and retrospectively angry. These feelings led us to consult with two other physicians, who recommended additional tests and who thought certain precautions were advisable (e.g., a stitch in the cervix).

Suzie's next pregnancy was a result of in vitro fertilization, which we chose because of our age (time had elapsed) and our difficulties conceiving. The birth of our twins followed seven months of bed rest, preterm labor, medication to control labor and prevent infection, constant monitoring, and several hospitalizations. Suzie went into labor in her 37th week, on the day that the medication was stopped, but her uterus ruptured. The babies' heartbeats could not be found, and they were delivered by emergency C-section. The situation was urgent and rushed, Suzie's belly being splashed with Betadine, which got into her eyes before she was knocked out. I was compelled to leave the operating room and stood alone down the hall in an adjacent unused space. Shaking like a leaf, I heard one doctor shout, "This one's not breathing!" When the obstetrician, Dr. Thomas, finally emerged about 30 minutes later to tell me both children were fine, I hugged her. (She later commented to Suzie, with some apparent wonder, "Your husband is *very* emotional!") Isaiah, the baby who was not breathing at first, was in the neonatal intensive care unit for three days. We observed and benefited from the remarkable attentiveness of the hospital staff. Isaiah quickly recovered and the members of our family were healthy for the next year.

However, when Judah, Isaiah's twin, was a year and a half he became precipitously and dramatically ill. Over a weekend, other members of the family had had a bad flu with a high fever. Judah seemed to have it as well, and we consulted with the doctors by phone. On Monday morning I took him to the pediatrician's office to be examined. The doctor found nothing exceptional, and I brought Judah home. I spoke with another member of the practice later that day because Judah's body had a reddish tinge and his hands and feet were cold; again I was told the symptoms were flu and fever related. The next day I came home at lunchtime to relieve Suzie, so she could go to work. Judah appeared listless and dehydrated, and we took him to the doctor again, although the office staff told us Judah could be seen only by a nurse practitioner.

Almost immediately on our arrival, the state of crisis was evident. Judah appeared to be failing rapidly. Different members of the pediatric practice poured into the consulting room. An ambulance was called and he was rushed to the Pediatric Intensive Care Unit at Lenox Hill Hospital. Within hours Judah was close to death.

He was diagnosed with toxic shock syndrome, exceedingly rare, especially in children. He was given antibiotics and his blood, heart, and lungs were carefully monitored. After about 24 hours his condition continued to worsen, as the oxygen level and the platelets in his blood were decreasing, and fluid was beginning to accumulate in his lungs. At a critical moment the doctors decided to move him from Lenox Hill to New York University Hospital, which had a larger pediatric ICU, more staff, and state-of-the-art life-support equipment. One of the chiefs of the NYU Pediatric Intensive Care Unit, Dr. Parnes, who lived five blocks from Lenox Hill, came to help transfer our son. The transfer was delayed for a while because Judah needed additional blood products (platelets and fresh frozen plasma) that were not readily available at Lenox Hill. Prior to the move, Parnes put a new, wider line into Judah's thigh, in anticipation of the several infusions and medications that would be needed. We then left, with the very competent and attentive paramedic telling the ambulance driver to go as fast as he could but to keep it steady. At about 10:00 Wednesday night, the ambulance sped down the East River Drive the 40 or so blocks from the first hospital to the second. I was told to travel separately and to go directly to the Admissions office to take care of the insurance information and the transfer, via computer, of the accumulated medical data.

When I rushed upstairs I found Suzie outside the PICU. She had been told to wait there while Dr. Parnes got Judah settled. When I arrived we impulsively went in and Parnes met us outside the curtained alcove in which Judah lay. He asked us to leave the PICU while he tended to our child. He was grave and very clear. Suzie asked him if Judah was going to live, and he said quite simply that Judah could die in a matter of hours.

Suzie and I waited in an empty shell of a room, with a few scattered phones and computers and chairs. We each, in our own crazed and anguished way, prayed. After about 20 minutes Parnes came out again to tell us that things were still not going well, that he was holding off intubating Judah for fear that it might lead to internal bleeding which could not be stopped. I called our pediatric practice and pleaded that one of our own doctors come immediately. Two were already on their way and arrived very shortly.

Forty minutes later we were told that Judah had been successfully intubated and we could see him. His small body lay motionless, hooked up to IV lines and machines. He was bloated from all the fluids that had spilled out of burst vessels into the body cavities. A medication was administered which kept him entirely paralyzed (to stop him from breathing against the respirator), and a heavy narcotic kept him totally sedated. He was given the most powerful antibiotics available and was receiving blood products. Doctors were pushing fluids through his system in an effort to flush out the toxin; he was also getting medication to sustain his blood pressure and his heart rate. All this was constantly monitored and adjusted.

Things were touch and go for several days, but Judah remained basically stable and further crises were averted. (The cause of one crisis—a resident changing a medication level—was identified by Suzie.) The medical team was keeping Judah alive while his body struggled to cope with the damage the toxin had caused. Lab results later revealed that the bacteria producing the toxin was a common staph bacteria found in all our bodies. For reasons unknown, Judah's immune system overresponded to the toxin by many factors of 10.

At one point, Suzie's brother Joe, a cardiologist on the West Coast, encouraged us to have Judah transferred to yet another hospital in the city. Based on information he had received, he told us that he thought the other hospital had a better PICU, and it had the only life-support machine in New York State which, if needed, could entirely reroute a patient's blood supply outside his body. My father, following a conversation with Joe, also wondered why we didn't have Judah transferred. He questioned why we weren't consulting with other doctors. At the time, however, Suzie and I were confident that Judah was receiving the best possible medical care, and we thought that he might very well not survive another transfer. Nonetheless we discussed this

option with Dr. Parnes, who assured us he had experience
with such transfers although he didn't deem one necessary
at that point.

Judah was on the respirator for eight days, but his body
rallied to emerge unharmed. When they took him off the
narcotic, he experienced withdrawal for about 36 hours,
during which he was intensely agitated, delirious, impossible to comfort, and unable to sleep. It wasn't until we took
him home several days later that he was willing to walk and
to smile. He remained tentative for a short while and was
more inclined than previously to focus obsessively on
holding small, cherished objects.

Several of Judah's PICU nurses and the ambulance
paramedic later told us how terrified they had been that
first night, how completely and effectively Dr. Parnes had
taken control, how direct and clear he was in giving orders,
carefully repeating them if needed. It was plain to us that he
(and they) had saved Judah's life.

During the two weeks he was in the hospital, Suzie and I
were both there during the day but alternated nights. When
things were relatively calm, we slept in a room set aside
down the corridor from the PICU, with other exhausted
parents—all of whom would leave their sleeping children
only with the nurses' assurance that they would be called if
the child awoke or there was any change in the child's status.
We were deeply impressed by the PICU staff, who regularly
encounter children on the verge of death. We knew we had
been very fortunate, more fortunate than most of the other
families who shared the PICU with us, many of whose children had chronic and incurable diseases.

A far less dramatic and threatening encounter with
doctors, but one that nevertheless had its impact on us,

occurred when I tore the anterior cruciate ligament in my knee playing touch football. The first doctor I saw, with an office in a very wealthy neighborhood and highly recommended by a physician-friend, suggested immediate surgery that would require a three-day hospitalization. Because he presented the situation as necessitating quick action, we were prepared to proceed with him until another friend, who had some knowledge of this particular doctor, advised us to get another opinion. So we got two. Doctors #2 and #3 counseled strongly against immediate surgery, given the swelling from the injury itself, and suggested physical therapy for several weeks prior to a proposed operation, to strengthen the muscles in the leg and facilitate postoperative recovery. They recommended an outpatient procedure, requiring no hospital stay. Doctor #1, prestigious and with a monumentally busy practice, appeared to be far less able than his colleagues.

Such were some of the experiences that lay behind us when Suzie and I encountered the discovery of my tumor one and a half years after Judah's illness. The abruptness, the shock, the overpowering disruption, being pulled out of expectations, safety, and security were familiar feelings, if necessarily muted in retrospect. With Judah's illness and with the miscarriages, I could readily recall traveling through the city from home to hospital as to a battlefront, cut off from my surroundings. We knew that chance, fortune and misfortune, could play a very significant role. One infectious disease physician had memorably remarked that the likelihood of a child's coming down with toxic shock syndrome was like that of a particular person being hit by a particular pigeon's shit as he walked the streets of Manhattan. Suzie and I knew that our attentiveness and vigilance were required and useful. We knew that accepting one expert's opinion might be hazardous. We were aware that there was tremendous variation among doctors in skill, wisdom, and reliability, and we were attuned to the very significant difference an individual doctor could make. We recognized that there could be substantial areas of the undetermined and unknown. While we didn't overtly reflect on any of this at the time, it played a part in how we approached the discovery of my tumor.

We relied heavily on our firsthand experience, we relied heavily on others, and I relied deeply on Suzie. At all the consultations to come Suzie asked significant questions and usually attempted to establish a more personal rapport with the doctors than I did. After each conversation with a physician, we reviewed our perceptions and understandings, and Suzie frequently remembered things that had been said that made a difference, things I had forgotten or dismissed. Her eyes and ears seemed to enhance my presence and identity (ever so slightly) and mitigate the impersonality of the proceedings and context. By her presence and through her questions and interjections, she brought into the doctor's immediate awareness the existence of our family. Often she provided the ballast necessary for me to hold a stable position, even one as simple as insisting that a doctor's presentation meet the minimum requirements of logic and common sense. Her presence steadied me in and out of the consultations, and at times when I couldn't bear being alone.

Chatter in the Infield

Two hours after I had been told of the tumor I entered my psychoanalyst's office for the first appointment following a five-week August vacation. The work I was doing in therapy was an elective extension of my training analysis. It was a peculiar, intense, human relationship—natural as anything we do and conceive, and constructed, bounded, contained (and thereby also similar to anything else we do and conceive). In my own experience of therapy, as well as in my work with patients, I wandered along a spectrum of possible locales—at times engaged with a powerful and direct questioner, a sharp-edged other, at times floating in the vicinity of someone much more diffuse. I sometimes imagined I was far more meandering, wayward, undisciplined, and lost than my principal interlocutor. At other times I knew better. There were many moments when, looking for certain kinds of interaction, for signs of struggle and conflict, for example, I failed to recognize the extensive intimacy of the interaction that was taking place. Craving contact, tolerating and seeking distance and difference, I walked along a water's edge. I would wade in and swim (reluctantly, eagerly), but in that autumn I was swept out by an undertow. Saul's office periodically provided me with something of a shore I returned to. It also served as a place where I reported my nightmares of drowning. And then, as well, it was a context in which we worked painstakingly and collaboratively toward constructing a raft that might help me to survive.

Sometimes Saul's office felt like a war room where maps were laid out and battlefronts plotted, a place where reconnaissance missions were conceived and their results reviewed, where strategy was outlined and scrutinized. It seemed as though I were repeatedly urged into an all-out battle, thoughtfully considered, for and by my self.

I began the September 9th meeting by saying to Saul, "Two hours ago I got some very bad news." We engaged in a very practical discussion. We gave detailed consideration to what I knew and understood, and what I didn't know and understand. Saul carefully questioned my thoughts and options and the alternatives that might exist. Our conversation, as at other times, promoted a more complete use of my experience and resourcefulness. At the end of the session Saul said, "Let your family warm you this weekend." A compassionate remark that, I sensed, came from personal experience. But not something I conceived as possible.

In those two hours between seeing Dr. Gibson and seeing Saul, I had called my parents and sister and my friend Eric. That evening I spoke with several other friends who are doctors (although their specialties were not oncology but gerontology and gynecology) and with my wife's brother (a cardiologist). An acquaintance, George, someone I had met socially once (his wife worked with mine), called to offer his help and experience; he was a psychiatrist who had worked as a liaison on a cancer unit for many years. Over the next few months I spoke with many of these friends and family very often, some almost daily. With this improvised community of listeners and observers, I reviewed every consultation I had, multiple times and in detail. Each review helped me to formulate questions, to gauge the risks and benefits of any proposed course of action, to understand information, to recognize the limits of what was known, and to pursue multiple options. Each person eased my being alone with life-and-death considerations and provided me with support, encouragement, and companionship.

Collectively, these friends, family, and colleagues sustained my efforts to make informed decisions amid immense uncertainty and pressure to act. While fostering careful inquiry into each medical issue, they also abetted my emotional separation from an individual physician's sphere of influence. The latter was perhaps most important: they freed me from concerns regarding too much dependence on any one doctor or any notions of loyalty to a specific physician.

I was quite fortunate to be able to engage this motley, devoted crew, particularly as it happened that my own internist and primary-care physician was away on vacation when I was informed of the tumor, and it was about a week and a half before he returned. When I finally was able to speak with him, it was as though the ship had already left the port, and I did not vigorously seek his input or advice. Still, quickly recognizing that my situation was very dangerous and complicated, he said, "I don't care how many opinions you get. I will write the referrals." This gesture was of considerable value as it diminished some of my immediate financial worries. It provided a bit of significant relief, although it did not allay my long-term concerns, as I knew that I did not have adequate life insurance.

My intermittent social reticence was *almost* transformed by having to deal with illness and facing death. For example, my initial response to George (the psychiatrist) was to say thank you, to be grateful for his generosity, but inwardly to assume that I would be reluctant to call him. Based on my prior behavior this would likely have been so. But fortunately, motivated by my life-and-death situation, I let myself rely on and use him and others in ways I formerly would not have found possible. I spoke with George in extended conversations, at times impatient with his methodical manner and yet simultaneously valuing and appreciating it.

George was one of the many doctors I talked with personally and not professionally. He was a medical strategist, someone I turned to for plotting and planning, and he was also attuned to the emotional impact of the unfolding events. George said to me at the outset that there would be days of good news and days of bad news and it was important to remind myself of this (and if I didn't, he would). His favorite and characteristic question was: "What will plan B be?" The question was often followed by: "What difficulties might we then encounter?" In a way that was comforting, he tended to use the first person plural as though we were in this together. Another of his mantras was that pursuing the best treatment was a process and while it might appear at times that there were simply contradictory options, these things usually sorted themselves out.

Like most of my friends and family, George was of the school that you don't stop looking until you're satisfied that you've arrived at the best available choice. While I was not inclined to settle, but rather to actively pursue each possibility, I know that I depended significantly on others' support and assurances that what I was doing made sense. Of course I was very clear that the responsibility and judgment were mine but, as I faced my endgame, many others were consistently available and provided sanctuary. So while the floor had been pulled out from under me, hands were stretched out for me to grasp, if only to stay suspended in midair. I reached out and seized several. On more than one social evening I apologized for my preoccupation but interrupted the flow of conversation several times to pose yet another question to a physician-friend. I trusted and found I would be indulged.

That first evening Suzie also talked to a very well known and highly respected pediatric ENT, who spoke with us as a courtesy to a mutual friend. Dr. Mills was held in immense esteem by everyone I spoke with. I suspected there was an added dose of appreciation because he had helped their children. His technical skill, clinical acumen, and personal manner were all lavishly praised. He generously offered to speak with us the next day, following our consultation and biopsy with Dr. Scheuer. Each of the doctors we spoke with that first evening thought a biopsy was in order, but none thought to caution me about where the biopsy should be done (in an OR), or whether it should be preceded by other tests, such as an MRI. It's possible these precautions were just assumed to be obvious and the doctors failed to recognize the extent of a layman's ignorance. It's also possible there was no commonly accepted medical practice, at least none that could be extrapolated from the information I provided.

What I *was* invariably cautioned about was the eccentric character and behavior of surgeons. It was the folk wisdom that in order to do what they do, surgeons had to be "cutting" when it came to personal interactions as well. Being disconnected, it was assumed, was a prerequisite for the specialty. Another piece of folk wisdom, borne out by my subsequent experience, was that each professional caste recommends and values itself above all others, although, even among other specialists, surgeons tend to dominate the hierarchy.

Also on that first evening, September 9th, I saw several of my own patients. I used as an excuse (for it did feel absurd) that I couldn't contact them in time to cancel, although, obviously, a note could have been left on my office door. The simple fact was that I wanted to see them, to minimize the disruption, to maintain normal activity (or the illusion thereof). I also wanted to be in contact with people I knew and cared about, with people who provided me with a sense of meaning and purpose. That night I even saw one patient for an initial consultation. In my mind there was a terrible threat to my continuity and the fabric of continuity between others and me. Not to talk about that felt incongruous, ridiculous. Yet the next morning I saw several more patients, again without revealing anything of my circumstances. I was fending off an insistent and intrusive anguish. I was fiercely uneasy and disoriented. And in the cocoon of my secret knowledge, I felt like I was bluffing.

No Dye

*O*n the afternoon of the second day, September 10th, my wife and I met with Dr. Scheuer, a prominent ENT surgeon. Our appointment was delayed because the films had been misplaced. When we were finally brought into the consulting room, Scheuer was preoccupied with an insurance matter of a prior patient, and this issue led to more than one disruption of our consultation, as he answered a receptionist who interrupted us with a question and then spoke with her again, having afterthoughts regarding the patient's payment method. As though in explanation, Dr. Scheuer mentioned that he was in the process of disengaging from my insurance company's network of providers.

It took him several minutes to focus. He began by putting up four sheets of film on the lightboard, a selection of the 17 sheets different from the ones I had been shown the previous day (that much I could tell). He noted that he was aware that I was a psychotherapist and made some remark implying that my profession probably made me better able to handle the news I had received the previous day. He then said jokingly and, it seemed, disjunctively, "I probably know more about you than you want me to know!"

Humorless and confused about what he meant, I responded, "I doubt that," inwardly registering my preference, which was that I wanted him to know *everything* about me. How could he know more than *I* wanted him to? What would I want to keep hidden from him? Perhaps he thought I could not tolerate his knowing how lethal the tumor was. Perhaps he knew more than *he* wanted to know.

Dr. Scheuer's opening remark went to the heart of a ubiquitous aspect of doctor–patient relations. Or the cliché thereof. The doctor—the one who knows (too much or too little), the patient—the one in the dark (uncertain if he wants to come into the light, doubtful if any light exists). Scheuer's comment touched on a prominent tension in all doctor–patient conversations, one that revolves around the hierarchical nature of the relationship and the knowledge and power differential between the participants. It pointed to the fundamental asymmetry in the interaction and the related struggles regarding openness and intimacy. In the moment, his remark served to unsettle me more than I had been—if that were possible.

Dr. Scheuer next asserted that a diagnosis would have been made easier if dye had been administered when the films were taken. I told him that I had been given the dye, had signed a release form for it, had had described to me the various side effects (a metallic taste in my mouth, flashes of warmth), had an IV inserted in my arm, and had seen and felt the nurse inject a fluid. The nurse had said at the procedure's conclusion, "I guess you're one of the lucky few who have no side effects from the dye." All indications were that it had been administered.

Scheuer then looked at all 17 sheets, one by one, each time announcing, "No dye! No dye!" After viewing each sheet, he handed it to Suzie. He told her how she should hold them, to "separate one group from another like a nursery school teacher." But there was no doubt in his mind about the absence of "contrast." (Scheuer, a prominent physician at a prestigious hospital, would prove to be wrong about this, although obviously I did not know it then, and I sought confirmation at several subsequent consultations. To no one else was there any question that dye had been administered.) Naturally, given my experience when getting the CT scan, I was bewildered and disturbed. When later that day I described Scheuer's evaluation of "no dye" to two of my friends who are doctors, they independently came up with the same idea that maybe I had been injected with water or a saline solution. They were unable to countenance that I had been injected with something else, or that Scheuer was simply wrong.

Dr. Scheuer rolled his eyes almost every time I conveyed one of Dr. Gibson's comments from the previous day. He disagreed, for example, with Gibson's judgment of the amount of destruction the tumor had already wrought; there was, he insisted, *no* significant erosion of bone. Unlike the preceding day, however, I now had my wife by my side. Like me, Suzie was unschooled in the art of x-ray interpretation, yet she quickly pointed out an area by my brain where there appeared to be a gap in the bone due to tumor intrusion. Scheuer grudgingly acknowledged that this could be the case.

He said he suspected that the tumor was benign and could be surgically removed, and then rapidly described the elaborate craniofacial surgery that would be involved. It would be performed by him and a neurosurgeon, with incisions at the top of my skull and the center of my face. Scheuer appeared intent on emphasizing the positive, on countering Gibson's gloom, and on moving the process along.

His next claim was consistent with this pattern. While he performed a physical exam (checking for loss of feeling in the face, weakening of my vision and hearing, and lumps in the lymph nodes, particularly of the neck, none of which had yet occurred), Dr. Scheuer asserted that there was no need for a biopsy at all: "Whether it's benign or malignant, it's got to come out." He noted that a so-called benign tumor can be very dangerous, particularly when it is located next to vital organs. He also argued that a biopsy could be inaccurate. It provided a sample of the tumor, but a tumor may not be consistent throughout, and the biopsied tissue might not be representative. A biopsy had its hazards as well. It could lead to a dangerous reconfiguring of the mass and precipitate bleeding that would be difficult to stop. Dr. Scheuer colorfully remarked that if he were administering the Board Certification Exams to someone in the relevant medical specialty and he described my case and asked, "Biopsy, yes or no?" and the candidate said that a biopsy *was* the next step, Scheuer would flunk him.

Dr. Scheuer contradicted Dr. Gibson on several other fundamental points. Dismissing several of Gibson's statements, he erupted at one point, "That's why *I'm* chairman of the department!"

Scheuer's reluctance to perform a biopsy confused me, and I questioned his reasoning several times. In response, after a few minutes, Scheuer reversed himself and agreed to do a biopsy. He then shifted the focus to where the biopsy would take place (in an operating room). He observed that, in any case, an MRI should precede a biopsy (as the latter could cloud the MRI results, which would reveal vascular structure better than a CT scan). He said he wanted the MRI performed at the hospital's tonier facility located elsewhere in the city because the radiography in the hospital was less reliable, as evidenced by the purported failure to administer dye in the case of my CT scan. He next wondered whether I actually wanted to make the additional trip that the two separate procedures (MRI and biopsy) would require. Baffled again by his thinking, I said I had no problem making two trips.

Dr. Scheuer's reversal of his strongly asserted position on a biopsy did not inspire confidence. It appeared to be less a matter of considered clinical judgment than a concession to the persistence of my doubt and inquiry. It was Dr. Scheuer's inconsistency that troubled me. Uncertainty is, of course, something entirely different, particularly when overtly acknowledged. But it was not a matter of admitted doubt here; in fact, Scheuer had been emphatically certain about things he later reconsidered.

Scheuer's general behavior and style were very disconcerting. In retrospect, it occurs to me that he probably thought he was acting in the interest of preserving my health. That is, he may have been eager to move the process along because of the urgency of my situation and before the delay that seeking other opinions might cause. Dr. Scheuer may have been gauging—and misperceiving—what kind of patient I was, namely, someone who was unlikely to act impulsively and for whom it was very important that his physician be calm and coherent. At the time, I had difficulty following Scheuer's explicit logic and it was impossible for me to make sense of what was implicit in his thinking.

Despite the troubling nature of the consultation, I left the encounter buoyed by the doctor's optimism. I preferred the feeling of hope and was initially almost celebratory. Just the night before, George had warned me that in consultations regarding cancer one must gird oneself for the roller coaster of good and bad news, but I was very much subject to the erratic dips and jolts of the moment. The qualities of the doctor's tone and presentation, his mood and manner, powerfully affected me.

I do not believe I was seeking an experience that mimicked the features and structure of an absurdist play. Yet Gibson, assuring me of his devotion, tried to convince me of the necessity of doing a biopsy on the spot, only to change his mind. He said the tumor had eroded significant tissue and bone and that my life was at stake. Then he gave me back my copay. Scheuer had thought not to do a biopsy and then changed his mind. He claimed no dye had been administered. He thought in a life-threatening situation I might not want to make an extra trip uptown. What there was of logic and accepted medical practice in all this eluded me. The Marx Brothers come to mind.

Eve's Offering

The sensation of living in an absurd drama was one reason I spoke with so many people and sought many different opinions. Doing so, I hoped, would widen the scope of my awareness and provide a means of checks and balances. While the knowledge base that sustains medical authority is far better established than ever before, the complexity and rapidity of medical progress, as well as the awareness of how mistaken medical consensus has been in the past, has led to what Sherwin Nuland recently referred to as a "spiral of uncertainty." There are simply no guarantees regarding the authority of any individual or institution.

I thus came to exercise an intense vigilance (although probably most aspects of the vigilance predated my illness). I wanted to clarify, clarify, and clarify, and then see if I could gain some small measure of lucidity. And I sought clarification most often about what seemed to be simple matters rather than technical ones I knew I wouldn't understand.

I recognized that some of the difficulties in my encounters with doctors were natural and inevitable. Neither the doctor nor I knew each other from Adam. Disturbing as it might be, my particular individuality was a very small factor, if one at all, in the doctor's mind. I was and often remained a virtual cipher. This was understandable given that, for many physicians, to engage with their patients in a genuinely personal manner is time-consuming and may be, in the physicians' judgment, only marginally "necessary." It might even be threatening and disturbing. Ostensibly it could foster unwanted intimacy or dependence and cloud a doctor's objectivity. Particularly when dealing with a life-and-death situation, a doctor might need to protect himself from attachment and the suffering that accompanies illness and death. By creating an aura of objectivity, a physician's detachment can provide both participants a semblance of security and comfort.

But the significant disparity between patient and doctor remains. While patients desperately yearn to trust their physicians and to hold them in the highest regard, the doctor is generally (if perhaps ambivalently) detached. While the patient hangs on the doctor's every word and gesture, the doctor stands back. In reaction to this common asymmetry, the many ways that patient and doctor respond to each other become covert or pro forma, part of a small, patronized sideshow.

In an initial consultation, where knowledge of each other is most obviously limited, there is almost always a dance like that on any blind date. It is unclear whether any connection will form, let alone whether the dancers will ever see each other again. There is thus the unacknowledged play of the doctor's wooing and the patient's romantic (or anti-romantic) proclivities.

Each doctor has a style intended to inspire trust. These styles are developed more or less consciously and are more or less effective. Some doctors I consulted appeared to rely on impressive furniture and institutional prestige, some on an apparent readiness to cut to the chase. Some relied on gruffness or on being casual, and some on giving the appearance of objectivity, although this stance was often construed and presented as an absence of affect. Some strove to give the impression that they couldn't care less if I became a patient of theirs. Others expressed an awareness of my predicament and exhibited compassion. But each style had a delicate measure of seductiveness.

Like other patients in a similar context, I was simultaneously discovering my illness, trying to educate myself about matters simple and complex, attempting to ascertain the boundaries of knowledge, and working hard to deal with the emotional freight of discussing something immediately life-threatening. I was also interviewing each doctor for a job. I was desperately searching for someone whose judgment appeared sound. I was evaluating the cogency of the physician's reasoning and assessing the depth of his or her clinical experience—and I was doing these things despite having very rudimentary medical knowledge. I was therefore also coping with the feelings of a child aware of his ignorance and unsure about the language being spoken, the assumptions, the conflicting possibilities and considerations.

Just putting on a hospital gown had an immediate and powerful impact on my sense of self. I expected that I would be submitting to procedures, cooperating and complying, permitting my body to be prodded and probed. While most of the talking was generally done after the examination, the gown and the procedures made it difficult to maintain any feeling of equality and led to a shift of status from which it was hard to recover.

All this helps to explain why it was exceedingly difficult for me to relate to a doctor as to another human being. Often it was just too much to countenance the physician's fallibility or self-interest. This was so despite my knowing that even the best doctors have flaws and vulnerabilities. I only gradually came to live with the idea that a doctor's personal and professional interests might conflict with mine in minor and significant ways. Such ways could be relatively obvious or subtle and hard to detect. A physician might find it very difficult to admit error or, like most of us, might simply be quite unaware of the various limitations of his thinking. He may believe he is the best despite indications to the contrary, or he may not believe he is the best but still thinks he is not obliged to refer a patient to someone better. These perceptions and sensations contributed to a situation in which I was constantly gauging, on relatively little evidence, who a doctor actually was.

Simultaneously, one tortuous emotional wave followed another. At every viewing of the films, when I saw the location of the tumor, its proximity to the optic nerves, the carotid artery, and the brain stem, there was the difficult process of orientation and then a renewed shock, like being waylaid and punched in the gut. There was then an extended scurry back toward the phantasm of equilibrium (or numbness). This would eventually be followed by yet another presentation of the stark danger in the images. After one consultation I might feel a resurgence of hope, an elevating sense that things might be manageable, even a giddiness, although this feeling came with its own caution. Following another I would be entirely shaken, terrified, plunged into a state of despair. I knew how much I wanted to hear certain things, and it felt almost impossible to sustain confidence in my presence of mind.

That there continued to be no symptoms enhanced the insecurity of perspective. It was all in my head. The tumor had had an entirely hidden and insidious onset. Of what value was the overt clinical picture? It had barely gotten me to the doctor in the first place and it had no correlation (fortunately and as yet) with the seriousness of the threat. It wasn't my intuition or any physical discomfort that told me my life was in danger. Amid such instability, the rigors of attention and reflection were my only option, and, paradoxically, trusting my own judgment became a necessity.

Awareness of my nakedness and the possibility of my imminent death sharpened my vision, my self-reliance, and my communion with other people. This was a seduction I could bite into.

Three Words He's Not Afraid to Say

*L*ate in the afternoon of Friday, September 10th (the same day I met with Dr. Scheuer), I spoke again with Dr. Mills (the highly recommended pediatric ENT), who graciously invited me to leave the CT scan films with the doorman of his building so that he could look at them over the weekend and call me. Over the next two days I waited anxiously to hear from him and I finally did, late Sunday evening. We had a five-minute phone conversation. Dr. Mills's description of the placement of the tumor and its proximity to vital organs was quite similar to Dr. Gibson's. He described a significant erosion of tissue and bone, the tumor's impinging on the cavernous sinus, and the strong possibility of its penetrating the bone that protects the brain in the area where it goes into the spine. He thought it likely that the tumor had also reached the dura, the membrane covering the brain. He described craniofacial surgery (a "relatively big surgery") in terms similar to Dr. Scheuer's. The soft tissue of the head and face would be "brought down and preserved"; brain contents would be retracted. He said he had spoken with a good friend and colleague, Dr. Barnet, with whom he had planned to play tennis the following morning. Dr. Barnet was, instead, planning to go in to his office at Memorial Sloan-Kettering to see me (among others). Dr. Mills said that Dr. Barnet was a great surgeon, the person who did the most surgery in this anatomical area in the country, if not the world. He said Dr. Barnet had done two or three such surgeries the previous week alone and added that Barnet could do in two or three hours what took other surgeons five or six.

Dr. Mills's words, and the arranging for the appointment the next day, emphasized the urgency of the situation and heightened my fear. I was trembling (and scribbling notes) during and after the conversation.

Almost immediately after hanging up the phone, although it was late Sunday evening, I called to cancel all my appointments for the following day. I responded to my patients' perplexity and their inquiries by stating that "something had come up" that necessitated the last-minute cancellations. If pressed further, I added that we could discuss their questions and the cancellation the next time we met. One patient later reported that she was frightened when she saw my name come up on her caller ID and had defensively reacted by being excessively businesslike.

On the morning of September 13th, four days after I first found out about the tumor, Suzie and I sat in Dr.

Barnet's waiting area, a clinic at Memorial Sloan-Kettering. Several of the friends (doctors) I had spoken with over the weekend had indicated that, given the circumstances, Memorial was probably "the place to be." It was the preeminent cancer center in New York, if not the world. It provided, if you believed their advertisements, the "best cancer care anywhere." There were, however, a few dissenting voices. People remarked that Sloan-Kettering was a very difficult place to work, that there were so many patients, all with cancer, that the hospital could at times be something like a factory. Research might take priority over individual patient care. I also was told that the doctors could be exceptionally arrogant, each assuming he or she was on Mount Olympus.

When I first heard these opinions I tended to dismiss them. I clearly didn't want to hear reservations about an institution I was looking to for care and security. I wanted to believe that I could rely on its authority, that these doctors would know, would be the best, and that I could trust in their experience and skill. So I was very prejudiced in his favor when Dr. Barnet greeted us, saying, "You must be the Newmans" (he told us we had been described as a "young couple").

Dr. Barnet is quite busy and isn't someone who appears to want to establish a personal or emotional connection. He attempts to be courteous but can be gruff, abrupt, and a bit edgy. He also tends not to establish eye contact. This eye-averted manner did not particularly bother me. I had repeatedly been warned, especially by other doctors, that surgeons are often personally cut off, a function of their work (and something which may have contributed to their choice of specialization). Dr. Barnet had come so highly recommended that I was eager to find him reliable, and on this first contact, any hesitations or misgivings I might have had were overridden. At some point toward the end of the consultation Suzie asked Dr. Barnet if he had children. It turned out that he had several, although his response to this simple question was hurried and perfunctory.

Dr. Barnet reviewed the films and recommended that a biopsy be done as soon as possible following the scheduled MRI. He presented himself as having a fiercely empirical stance. "It could be any of 40 different tumor types, and I will make no assumptions until after a biopsy. I won't even discuss the possibilities." At two points he emphatically said, "There are three words I am not afraid to say: *I don't know.*" Although the declaration was definitely rhetorical (it was clear from the delivery that he had uttered these exact words a multitude of times), it nonetheless appeared honest, was inoffensive, and was in keeping with my preferred style and prejudices. At first glance, Dr. Barnet's attitude stood in sharp contrast to Dr. Scheuer's. So, primarily on the basis of Dr. Mills's exalted recommendation, I arranged to have Dr. Barnet perform the biopsy in an operating room at Memorial Sloan-Kettering four days later (following an intervening MRI). During the procedure a frozen section would be taken: a sample of the tissue that was removed would be sent on the spot to the pathology lab for immediate testing and a preliminary reading of the pathology. We could thus expect more information on that very day.

The MRI was performed at the midtown facility, and I made sure to get an extra set of films. (It took me weeks to get a second set of the initial CT scan.) Before the biopsy I conferred by phone with another physician, Dr. Logan, who had been recommended by several sources. He too was an ENT surgeon; he had worked at Memorial for more than a decade and was now a prominent surgeon in head and neck oncology at Beth Israel Hospital. He agreed that a biopsy was the preferred course.

Whose Pathology Is It?

*O*n the day of the biopsy, Suzie, my parents, and my sister all came to the hospital. I had been told the procedure would last about one hour. Outside the OR I gave Dr. Barnet the MRI films, which he said he would run upstairs to look over with the radiologist. Lying on a gurney outside the OR, I saw him hurriedly glance at a couple of sheets, holding them up to the ceiling lights, as he left.

Hours later I woke up in the recovery room, with some difficulty breathing. Suzie soon came through the swinging doors to my right. She had asked to see me and been told she could do so for one minute, after which she would have to wait until I was moved to another holding area. On seeing her I immediately asked if she knew the results from the frozen section. Suzie said she didn't know. But she did. Dr. Barnet had spoken with her, my parents, and my sister directly after the biopsy. He had informed them that the results from the preliminary pathology revealed that the tumor was malignant and inoperable. He said it could be treated with chemotherapy and radiation, although his manner was grave and forceful and did not prompt hope or optimism. Nonetheless, out of concern for me coming out of the anesthesia and from fear at what she had heard, Suzie indicated to me that she didn't know.

Later, in a secondary recovery room, Suzie apologized for not having been forthright and conveyed Dr. Barnet's remarks. We waited several hours for him to return to speak with me. In the interim my other family members each spent some time with me, all with a sad, anxious, and morbid air but trying nonetheless to distract me. As I was still a bit woozy from whatever medication they had given me, I felt only mildly perturbed and mostly numb.

When Dr. Barnet arrived hours later, with a resident in tow, he spoke curtly, as though he had no time to spare. He looked exhausted. While I was still a bit groggy from the anesthetic, Dr. Barnet informed me of the results of the preliminary pathology findings, "*As I had thought,* the tumor is too extensive for surgical resection." (Even in such circumstances, I did not appreciate his unnecessary "as I had thought.") "It is an adenocarcinoma," he continued, "a malignant and potentially aggressive tumor, with its origin probably in the salivary glands in the nose. Chemotherapy and radiation should begin as soon as possible. I have informed my receptionist, and when you get home she may already have left you a message regarding appointments at the beginning of next week with the medical and radiation oncologists. You can go ahead and have the appointments even *before* the final pathology results, which should be available in three workdays." Barnet spoke with an air of authority, seriousness, and urgency, and without qualification.

His brief comments were terrifying. They did not invite any discussion; apparently there was no point. What I had understood earlier as his uncertainty now seemed transformed into emphatic conviction. The tone of profound urgency, the lack of a surgical option, and the absence of any communication regarding the possible effectiveness of the other treatments felt like a death sentence, which, even through my numbness, I could still understand.

On the very gloomy way home from the hospital, there was a moment when I felt such intense pressure on my bladder that I asked to stop the car and got out to pee on the street behind a parked car. The doorman from a nearby building came out to scream and curse at me. The resulting sense of humiliation and embarrassment became a common feeling in the subsequent weeks. It arose from so many things being entirely out of my control—as was the feeling of my being on the far side of a dividing line separating the living and the near dead.

There was no message on the answering machine when I arrived home, so I waited over the weekend to find out when my next appointments would be.

On Monday morning, September 20th, I spoke with Dr. Barnet's receptionist, Alice, who said she was unaware that she was expected to make any appointments. I stressed what I understood from Dr. Barnet to be the urgency of the situation.

Alice contacted me the following afternoon to inform me of appointments with the radiation oncologist, Dr.

Hughes, and the medical oncologist, Dr. Samuel, but for several weeks later. I said that wasn't soon enough, according to Dr. Barnet, and she responded by noting that, if I wanted appointments sooner, "Dr. Barnet would have to get involved." I agreed with her and asked her to get Dr. Barnet involved.

Having inspired in me a tremendous sense of urgency (he had said I should proceed with the appointments even before Wednesday, when the biopsy results could be expected), Dr. Barnet appeared to have absented himself.

That I was left adrift in regard to my further appointments may seem trivial. But it added to my sense of powerlessness and vulnerability. Any serious illness can lead to feelings of being peripheral and expendable, but this is only reinforced by a doctor's oversight or inaccessibility. Under some circumstances it may be possible to be philosophical about physician fallibility, but as a fragile patient I felt there was no margin for error by the doctor or by me.

I spoke with two of my friends who were physicians, one of whom contacted Dr. Samuel directly while the other called Dr. Barnet. Obviously doctors can get through where patients can't, and this form of advocacy brought me much earlier appointments. Following his conversation with Dr. Barnet, my friend George conveyed to me that he had considerable respect for him, that he seemed very knowledgeable, and that other physicians he had spoken with also thought Barnet "first-rate."

As the next few days passed, the final biopsy results from the pathology lab were still not available. However, Alice assured me several times that this was nothing unusual (although my physician-friends thought otherwise). I believe that I was fairly successful containing my anxiety, but Alice still sounded curt and impatient. Over the course of two long weeks I called a couple of times, always restrained and deferential.

It was typical for me to be more reserved than insistent, careful not to be imposing or offensive. Under the circumstances I pushed these attitudes slightly aside; they became close to inconsequential. They *almost* didn't matter; I *almost* didn't care. But I still did not want to appear to be a pest (even though it was my life that hung in the balance). I was still concerned that my seeking other opinions would be judged harshly as disloyalty and distrust. At one point during the two-week period of waiting for the pathology results, Suzie and I came to Memorial to gather the folder of original films to present for another opinion, and I was sent from one office to another, finally running into Dr. Barnet. I was basically mute; I failed to say a word to him about my distress with the appointment making or the delay in regard to the pathology. I was wary about conveying frustration, impatience, or disaffection.

Of course, many doctors are exceedingly busy, overburdened in ways both within and outside their control. But the demands on a doctor's time and attention, generally quite evident, can exacerbate patients' feelings of dependence. The patient senses that he needs the doctor far more than the doctor needs him. It is also commonly the case that a doctor meets with a patient only a few times, or discontinuously and rarely, and there is little motivation and almost no room for open discussion of the personal interaction. Patient advocates may bemoan the fact that many patients continue to treat physicians as deities, but there are deep structural and emotional reinforcements to the patient's role as supplicant.

Yet the figments and fragments of my inhibition were gradually being overcome by an awareness of a piercing, relentless, supervening self-interest. I sought to be internally almost ruthless in my scrutiny of the medical care, while also being cautious, considered, and diplomatic. My character "pathology," especially my restraint, was present but yielding. The lab had still not issued a report on the tumor's.

An Orderly Inquiry

Although I did not know it at the time, my conversations with the first trio of physicians (Gibson, Scheuer, and Barnet) were only a beginning, a mere initiation into what some people call "the consultation process." This three-word phrase, however, misleads as it dignifies, for it appears to contain and rationalize what was often a helter-skelter, fortuitous, traumatic series of events and encounters.

It was in the face of such quasi-chaos that I saw many doctors. The more I encountered confusion and a divergence of opinion, the more that needed to be clarified—if it could be. The less hopeful and certain the treatment options, the greater the need for confirmation or for another perspective—if there was one.

So I spread the net widely and received a variety of names that required some sorting. I evaluated the referrals first by their sources—my respect for the individuals making the referrals, their knowledge and reliability, their closeness to the recommended doctor. I also tried to corroborate referrals by asking others.

Two or three times I was given the name of a doctor who turned out to be someone just outside the specialties relevant to my case. Generally, though, I followed through on almost every avenue suggested. I went to some consultations even when I thought beforehand it was unlikely I would ultimately use those doctors.

I did not assume any doctor or institution had a monopoly on knowledge or expertise. Reputations are like caricatures: some sharply drawn, others flimsy and false. To have a semblance for evaluating, I had to meet with the person in whom the reputation was vested. If there was a way of knowing, I had to be in the presence of the doctor myself. But regardless of the tension and my impressions, I benefited from every encounter, for each one provided me with further education, greater familiarity with the various options, and more awareness of the areas of disagreement and uncertainty. There was a quantitative, as well as qualitative, aspect to this: accumulated experience added up to a more refined ability to make distinctions.

Inquiry into the illness also involved some inquiry into its etiology. Of course it had occurred to me that the environment, in one form or another, might very well have played a significant role in the development of my cancer. In particular, as I am an artist as well as a therapist, it worried me that the materials I had used (paints, varnishes, mediums, stains), which were often noxious, were also toxic. At each consultation I would ask about the possible genesis of the tumor, and I uniformly received a shrug of the shoulders and a statement that the doctor had no idea. Similarly, I would ask how long it was thought the tumor had been growing in my head, and the medical shoulders would rise again. "Two years? Five years? No idea." During the course of its existence, a tumor could, apparently, change its rate of growth. I found out on the Web and from several physicians that there was one study indicating that workers exposed to wood dust over several decades had an increased tendency to develop adenocarcinoma in the naso-pharynx, but no one thought this finding applicable to me.

Several people had also begun to talk to me about alternative medicine, yoga, meditation, and diet. Often their suggestions were a measure of what they took to be the hopelessness of my situation. (Just as some people thought it encouraging to tell me stories about an aunt who had been told to go home and buy her burial shroud and, lo and behold, she was still around to irritate the family 10 years later.) I would thank them but note that at this moment I was not pursuing alternatives to conventional medicine. Because of the size and location of the tumor, I felt that I did not have the time such means would require.

My response was similar when others encouragingly murmured about how important my attitude was, as though I could shrink the tumor by believing I could do so. While I am quite respectful of the forces of mind and mind–body interdependence, I was not inclined to place my bets on these methods. The implicit logic, when reversed, could hold me responsible for my condition.

I *was* in imminent danger. But when people would bring up experimental treatments ("Ask about monoclonal antibodies!") I would say, "I'm not there yet." I did not by any means rule out such treatments, but I felt an urgency to pursue first what conventional medicine had to offer. This was my immediate, primary focus, obviously reflecting my priorities and beliefs. I was aware that the medical establishment, like any other, could be insular and wrong. Egregious historical examples came to mind: the blaming of parents for autism and schizophrenia and, more pertinent to surgery, prefrontal lobotomy for all manner of mental disorder in the 1940s and 1950s. But I wanted to know the extent of our present medical and scientific knowledge as it pertained to my illness, and this project in itself obliged me to pursue a careful, orderly inquiry. Given the intensity of my anxiety, I did not describe things to myself in this fashion. I felt more like a leaf in the wind for whom order signifies nothing.

The ferociously variable gusts blowing me about were accelerated in the atmosphere that surrounded each doctor's office. So Suzie and I developed a bit of a comic routine that facilitated *our* rounds. Every visit to a physician involved about 45 minutes of travel each way and then one and a half to two hours of waiting beyond our appointment time (this was New York). We would finally be ushered into a consultation room and then often wait an additional 20 to 30 minutes. Despite this consistent delay, it was my nature to show up for the appointments when they were supposed to occur. I imagined we were seen in some relation to the time we showed up and our scheduled appointment. When we were at long last brought into the doctor's office, and he or she was still not present, we would play with the idea that the doctor was hiding, or invisible, or had shrunk to a minuscule size, and we began to address the physician nonetheless. Mostly this game led to a lot of giggling until the moment of the doctor's entrance.

The Putting Out of Eyes

On September 23rd, 14 days after the flood waters began rising, I saw Dr. Satlovski, a medical oncologist at Mount Sinai. I had been told by one physician that the team at Sinai was too surgically oriented. Yet I had also been told by George that Dr. Snow, who ran the oncology department, was excellent, and George strongly recommended my consulting with the Sinai team.

Dr. Satlovski is Russian and I found his English difficult to understand. On many occasions I had to ask him to clarify what he had said, and I periodically gave up. My difficulty in comprehension impeded and curtailed the proceedings, and the doctor appeared more impatient and jittery than he might have otherwise. Despite his gentleness and thoroughness, I could not speak with him effectively or gauge the qualities of his thinking. While the barrier of the doctor's accent was, for me, insurmountable (and quite concrete), it felt like only a very particular instance of the more general, ubiquitous struggle for comprehension.

The language difficulty was analogous, for example, to the problems I had on the phone. With almost every doctor I saw, our in-person consultation was followed by phone conversations: if I had further questions, if we were waiting for test results, if there were new recommendations based on new information or further discussion with colleagues.

These phone contacts were a whole other arena of intense anxiety and stress. I very often was waiting for a phone call or for several calls. I borrowed Suzie's cell phone, which I had never used, and it became essential: the last thing I wanted was not to be available when a doctor finally called. (Once I was contacted by a doctor while I was driving on the West Side Highway and pulled over and searched for my sheet with questions; once I was shopping in a large pharmacy and found a quiet aisle.) I was always concerned that I be prepared for such phone conversations— as aware as I could be of what my questions were and able to pursue my difficulties in understanding what was being communicated. On the phone my apprehension and tension were heightened as there was less opportunity to let things sink in and to respond or inquire.

On the same day as my visit with Dr. Satlovski, the medical oncologist at Mount Sinai, I had my initial consultation with Dr. Hughes, a radiation oncologist at Sloan-Kettering. We were, at the time, proceeding on the premise that the pathology of the frozen section was accurate. Dr. Hughes explained to me how she would plan the radiation. Owing to recent technological advances and accumulated clinical experience, it is now possible to exercise significant control over the amount of radiation that is delivered to every point of a tumor. Based on data from CT scans and MRIs, a computer generated three-dimensional model can be constructed. Given the location of my tumor, the obvious primary concern was how much radiation the adjacent vital structures could tolerate. The principal worry was the impact on the brain stem and my eyes—the nerves to the eyes and the optic chiasm. Dr. Hughes said that, because of the aggressiveness of the tumor, she was going to use a dose higher than what was generally thought to be tolerated by these structures. Damage to the eyes might not be evident for some time; it was possible, for example, that I could go blind several years down the road. I said then (and would repeat this to other doctors in other contexts, generally with a choked voice) that my life was far more important than my sight. I reiterated this emphatically.

I know this is not something anyone could say easily; like others, I treasure my sight. In particular, as a painter I have an intensely passionate relation to what I see and make. I care deeply when I look; the slightest variations, the subtlest shifts of color, value, placement, gesture draw my attention and appear meaningful. But I never doubted the relative value of my eyesight. A neuroophthalmologist whom I saw months later adeptly referred to this aspect of the decision making as a "no-brainer."

Dr. Hughes, in her mid to late 50s, was cordial, warm, and unassuming. She readily established a casual and friendly tone. A resident accompanying her initiated the interview and handled some of the more rudimentary questions.

Hughes said that, given the diagnosis, we stood only about a 50–50 chance of being able to eliminate the tumor. Her tone was nonetheless (and incongruously) upbeat and reassuring. She described the process of preparing for the radiation. We would schedule a "simulation" as soon as possible. This was a procedure in which a molded mask made of plastic mesh, would be made of my head. The mask would be used to hold me in place by being clamped to a base on the table while the radiation was administered. Being placed in the exact same position every day was critical for controlling the quantity and direction of the radiation. The fixed orientation on the table would also be accomplished by placing several small but permanent tattoo dots on my face.

Dr. Hughes described the anticipated side effects of the radiation. These included burnt skin around my nose and eyes, burning and sores on the interior of the nose and mouth, a substantial decrease in saliva, loss of appetite, congestion, some hair loss, headaches and severe fatigue. The simulation was scheduled very soon (with some advocacy by Dr. Hughes), for the following Monday, September 27th. A dental checkup and a hearing test were to take place on the following day. The dental appointment was to evaluate whether or not I would need a special mouthpiece to be used in conjunction with the mask and also to establish a baseline, as the radiation would negatively affect my teeth and gums. Urine collection (over a 24-hour period) was scheduled as well, this in preparation for my appointment with the medical oncologist, Dr. Samuel. The radiation and the chemotherapy needed to be coordinated, as they are often done in concert, and certain chemotherapies sensitize tissue to radiation, so that the latter needs to be adjusted and calibrated accordingly.

Following our appointment, Suzie and I were despair-
ing. Fifty–fifty did not sound like very good odds. Suzie
said to me then, as she would several times subsequently,
that there was no reason why I shouldn't be in the 50% (or
10% or 20%) that survive. At least there was no reason that
we knew of. All the numbers that were cited had to be
contextualized: Did they apply to someone of my age and
general well-being, treated by this particular doctor at this
particular institution? With this size tumor, with this pathology, in this location? It was clear we were dealing with
very rough estimates. In my initial review of some articles
on the Internet, I found it exceedingly difficult to identify
studies that were pertinent or pertinent enough. What I did
find I had a hard time wading through. The pathology of
the tumor, its size and location, the treatments attempted,
the years of follow-up—there were often too many variables and too few correlations with my condition for me to
make use of the information. That many of the figures
were terrifying made it virtually impossible for me to sort
out the data effectively (or so it then seemed; in retrospect,
the information was quite grim and clear enough). I also
knew that research and treatments change rapidly and that
what I was reading may well have been the case two years
ago but might no longer pertain to the present.

Therefore, while I agreed with Suzie and would place
my hope in being among those that survived, I also
strongly heard the risk and the danger. A friend teased me
that a psychotherapist could lose several of his senses and
still be able to work. Taste, touch, sight, smell. I counted
them up, reviewed them, and imagined losing one or two
or three.

Traffic

O n the day following the meeting with Dr. Hughes, Friday, September 24th (15 days after I spoke with Dr. Gibson), I saw Dr. Logan at Beth Israel for an initial consultation. I had spoken with him by phone a week earlier about the advisability of a biopsy (which he had encouraged me to have, as scheduled, at Memorial). Dr. Logan, who appeared to be around 50, was born in the Midwest and has a gentlemanly manner. He is attentive and calm and takes his time.

After reviewing the films and examining me, Logan was somber and direct. He carefully stated that his remarks were provisional, pending the final outcome of the pathology. If the tumor were an adenocarcinoma, then a lot would depend on whether it was low or high grade—that is, how infiltrative it was and how rapidly it was growing. Dr. Logan expressed the feeling that, because of where the tumor was located and because I had a minor symptomatic response, the tumor might well be on the low-grade side of the scale (after all, my eyesight had not been affected, nor were the feelings in my face or my hearing; I didn't have headaches). Logan's tone conveyed, however, that he was skeptical that the tumor *was* low grade. He clearly didn't want to hold out false hope or be inappropriately optimistic. Prefacing his further remarks by saying he preferred being blunt given I was a man with a lot of responsibilities, three young children and patients of my own, Dr. Logan stated that if the tumor were high grade I might have only a 10% to 20% chance of surviving two years. In other words, I might die quite soon. Unable to skirt cliché, he said he thought I should get my affairs in order.

Logan had the impression that the tumor was inoperable, but he wanted it to be discussed at Beth Israel's weekly tumor board meeting the following Tuesday (four days later). He was going to be out of town, but he introduced us to Dr. Bloch—whom I had also heard of as being a sterling surgeon—and said that Bloch would be covering for him and we should speak the following week after the tumor board meeting. Logan also asked if other parts of my body had been scanned and then recommended that I have a CT scan of my lungs to check for metastases. This scan was scheduled for that afternoon by his staff. He said that with a tumor of my type, cancer generally spread first to the lymph nodes in the neck and then to the lungs. It was the latter metastases that were likely to be fatal.

Suzie and I left the office stunned again. No matter what we had been told in the past, each new encounter, each consultation, could bring us back in touch with the reality of the situation. Check for metastases to the lungs. A 10% to 20% chance of surviving two years. It was hard to sustain acute awareness of the danger. Such a response may have been natural, protective, and adaptive, but it led to feelings like vertigo, to a dizzying, stumbling, instability. The oscillation itself fostered a numbness, as one becomes inured to successive shocks.

Following the appointment, Suzie was going home and I was going to the CT scan facility when we got stuck in traffic. I suggested we get out of the cab and walk, and inattentively opened the door in the midst of a densely crowded street (Third Avenue in the 20s) where I thought the cars were stopped. I then proceeded to drop the folder containing the films and, with the cabbie screaming at me and cars honking and screeching, retrieved them.

No Dye, Again

The CT scan facility was a depressing place, as most waiting rooms are. There was a patient loudly using the receptionist's phone to do business. There were very young children. At the time I was trying to read Don DeLillo's *Underworld,* a large heavy book I lugged around, able to read only a paragraph or two before my mind drifted. (I eventually gave up on the idea of being able to read.) The beginning of the book, with a description of a game at the Polo Grounds, had a dazzling trompe l'oeil effect, but I lost interest.

When I was finally brought into the imaging part of the facility and lay down on the table, the technician asked if I had ever had a CT scan before. I said, "Yes, as a matter of fact, just a few weeks ago, when I was told I was being injected with dye, although apparently I wasn't." He thought for a moment and responded, "Oh, I guess that happens sometimes." He then indicated that there would be no such concern today as no dye would be injected. I had heard Dr. Logan order the scan with dye and had carried the instructions with me to the facility (and read them), so I knew the technician's remark to be incorrect. I said, "But Dr. Logan ordered the scan to be done with dye." The technician answered, "But Dr. Vitarelli, the radiologist, says it doesn't have to be." I said that I assumed Dr. Logan had ordered the dye for a reason. The technician then asked me to get up from the table and have a seat. He went into an adjoining room and returned moments later to report that Dr. Vitarelli had reiterated that the dye was not necessary. I said I would like Dr. Vitarelli to speak to Dr. Logan before we proceeded. The technician again retreated to the adjoining room, from which he reappeared just a few moments later. "Dr. Vitarelli says if you want dye, you can have dye."

Unwritten Letters

*M*uch of what went on in my mind (or, more accurately, in my entire body) I don't want to recall. There are states of being that accompanied me that I prefer not to reenter. No matter what I did, inevitably, the possibility of my dying was soon right before me, around me, within me. I would think of not experiencing the pleasures of life, of missing being with my children and Suzie, of her dealing with things without me, and I would have to stop thinking. While it was almost always I who would bring up the subject of my death, Suzie did say to me a few times, "Every night I'd be waiting for you to come through the door."

In the weeks following my diagnosis there was an extended period during which each time I did anything, it occurred to me that it could be almost the last time: giving my children a bath; putting them to bed; seeing; touching. With each person I spoke to, I wondered if I would never talk with him or her again or I imagined having only a few months of further contact. There was an aura of imminent loss that surrounded and terrified me. I tried reasoning with myself in several directions, but I could not tolerate conceiving of leaving the people I love.

Yet there were also moments (very few) when I thought I could live with dying—although such acceptance (coerced, as it was) seemed demented.

I began composing letters to my three children, letters I thought could be read at different moments in the future. I returned frequently to putting together words to my nine-year-old son:

Dear Jacob,

I am writing this with the understanding that I will not be around at times I would like to be, for you and for me. When you want to play (always), when you accomplish things, when you want to talk with me, when you don't but I do . . . I would like to write something that could feel like a hand on your shoulder or a teasing jab in your gut . . . or an embrace . . . .

But such words carried a weight they could not bear. (Besides my being unable to find a consistent tense to write them in.) The words embodied an unrealizable request: listen to me, be with me, comfort me. I wanted to feel that I would continue to matter. I wanted to comfort and console him. I wanted to prepare him and provide for him. I wanted to tell him what I knew, had learned, thought I understood. I wanted to survive. The imagined letters failed to lessen the terror and isolation and just intensified the pain.

So I never got further than the opening lines or a stray fragment. I came to think that such letters could be written only when it was finally clear to me that I had almost no time left. Then, I imagined, I would overcome the pain of imminent absence. I would easily resurrect the hurtful thoughts and feelings and bring them back to life—if I couldn't bring myself. Then, in the midst of relinquishing attachments, writing might provide me with some relief.

Like a trick candle, I sometimes revive the experience of being enflamed and sometimes of being permanently snuffed out.

Parallel Parking

*I*t was simply too painful to imagine my complete and permanent absence. While I felt some of the depth and intensity with which it would be experienced by those close to me, I knew and appreciated that life goes on. I could imagine, with a mixture of pain and gratitude, my children experiencing joy, even in my absence. There was the feeling, though, that to all but a very few, I was inessential and dispensable. A reality, but not one ordinarily so prominent. When I wasn't talking with doctors, or talking about my talks with doctors, I was imagining leaving the people I love.

Such thoughts, however natural and inevitable, became too disturbing, and, on Sunday, September 26th, in an uncharacteristic gesture, I decided to avoid them—if possible, to

67

stop them when they began, or at least to prevent them from being elaborated in any way. I had tolerated the thoughts, even permitted their flourishing, for a little more than two weeks. But the feelings were too acute. That explains to me the necessity of the censoring gesture, my unexpected ability to enact it, and its substantial success.

It was something I had never before attempted. In fact, facing the grimmer side of experience and history had always struck me as obligatory and essential. Not *wanting* to think about something had never seemed much of an argument for not thinking about it. I was always concerned that any limited prohibition of thought tended to widen out ("You can't hold down one thing without holding down the adjoining"). I recognized that more horrors go on than I could know, but acknowledging the gruesome parts of life, past and present, seemed a necessary means for living fully. I positioned myself on the side of admitting weakness and against romanticizing, glorifying, making pretty, censoring. I resisted contemporary impulses toward mythology as being far more confining than revelatory.

Therefore, limiting what I imagined, censoring my thinking, felt implausible. But it speaks to an earlier failure of my imagination to encounter consciously, fully, and closely enough a psychic pain I could find no means of tolerating and which therefore required conscious suppression. The deliberate censorship was a victory for the defense.

I remember talking with Eric, a friend, about some of these things in his car on the way to and from his daughter's soccer game. I think this conversation was pivotal in my making the decision to ban such thinking. I appreciated his saying that he had imagined my death and my family without me: "I've thought about how I would try to stop by on my way home from work." I recall holding back my tears as we arrived and got out of the car, the children leaving the back seat. I see the field, the sun and shadows, the places we sat, the position his daughter played (right fullback), the high reeds beside the field. I remember Eric's excursion to get lunch. It is intriguing why all this landscape comes back to me. Perhaps it was my sharply heightened sense of vulnerability. It was an unusual circumstance—we were tagging along, attending his child's soccer game. Eric's daughter had that day a school friend visiting her as well, so no doubt our plans to see each other were last-minute. Also, perhaps unexpectedly, my nine-year-old son was perfectly amenable to the circumstances. The feeling that I was in something of a cocoon, cut off from my surroundings, paradoxically intensified the sharpness of the light, the darkness of the shadows, and their visual impact on my memory.

It may have been that same weekend, or a bit later, that, lying in bed with Suzie, I said, "I'm going to say this only once . . . and perhaps it's unnecessary . . . but if I do die . . . if you do find someone you love . . . I want you to have that." On yet another occasion, and despite my above disclaimer (about speaking of this only once), I remarked, "Whatever happens, I know you won't be able to find someone who can parallel park like I can."

Something Is Wrong with You

*I*n the standard medical model, a doctor assumes a posture which is supposed to entail minimal interpersonal complications. But in psychotherapy the relationship between patient and therapist, including all the complications, is the means of the process. It is a principal subject, a primary vehicle of therapeutic action, and the arena in which and through which development and change occur.

Of course, the therapist's reserve can resemble and might be identified with the comportment of a medical doctor. There are historical roots that join the two professions, and similar concerns justify the reserved demeanor. A common value is the sustained focus on the patient and a subordination of the healer's desires to the patient's interests. Yet within psychotherapy there are also traditions that have long recognized the complicated crosscurrents of interpersonal influence, and thus the inconsistencies, which result from the posture of reserve.

In fact, a prevalent contemporary view of psychotherapy embraces the understanding that both participants are vulnerable and reactive to each other. There is an enhanced appreciation that both patient and therapist have desires for recognition and admiration and that the therapist's self-interest, often unconscious, may always be active. There is, in general, an increasing tendency to acknowledge the impact of the practitioner's subjectivity, as well as the fact that there can be reciprocal impulses to collude or manipulate and coerce.[1] This view has had, in some respects, a withering impact on the therapist's authority, although now the potential on both sides for evasion, for seduction and abandonment, is mined for its therapeutic possibilities. Alongside rigorous and detailed inquiry into the patient's motivation, there is a focus on the vicissitudes and dynamic meanings of the therapist–patient relationship, as expressed in both parties' words and actions and internal experience.

Prior to the period of my illness, my work as a therapist involved encouraging intimacy and fostering attachment and meaningfulness in the relationship. It also involved relatively rare presentations of aspects of my personal circumstances and history, presentations that ran counter to the therapist's general reserve. A premise, however, was that all interactions, to varying degrees, revealed my subjectivity.

This approach is not without its contradictions. The more impersonal aspects of the relationship—the limited time, place, and frequency of the meetings, and those features which clearly serve the therapist's interests (payment, restricted access)—inevitably clash with the personal and intimate qualities. As my patients point out, much of our encounter is at my discretion (despite my being a hired hand). I set overt boundaries in numerous ways, including limits on my participation. There is a very significant disparity between patient and therapist in what is revealed and acknowledged. Along with engagement and intimacy, there is a deliberately fostered detachment. The process of therapy draws on this inconsistency of deep personal involvement being constantly enacted within a structure that distances and protects, and thereby fosters scrutiny of the relationship.

My earlier experiences with illness and with my clinical work during those periods had marked me very personally, and therefore as a therapist as well. The miscarriages and Judah's illness considerably added to and altered my experience of patienthood and its intense vulnerabilities. In those instances, I had returned to work very quickly, still raw and isolated. I kept my experiences mostly private and, as a result, felt remote. Retrospectively, I was bothered by what had felt like my own emotional unavailability, my buried feelings, and I held myself partially responsible for the lack of patients' inquiries into my absences. It was earlier in my professional life when I was more tentative and restrained, although the experiences with illness led me to reconsider some of my insulating behavior.

These many attitudes informed my cancer dialogues with the doctors. They encouraged a sensitivity to the contributions of both the physician and the patient (i.e., me) to what happened between us. They also helped to shape the context in which I worked with my patients and into which my tumor abruptly intruded.

All the medical appointments made it necessary for me to cancel many therapy sessions, immediately raising the question of what I communicated to patients about my illness and about my plans. Within a week or so I became aware that quite soon I would likely have to discontinue meeting altogether, as whatever the treatment was—surgery, chemotherapy and/or radiation—it would necessitate a medical leave at the very least. But there was a tremendous amount of uncertainty about the treatment, its duration, when I would need to stop working, if and when I would be able to return, and, of course, what the diagnosis and prognosis (and outcome) would be. Particularly given the degree of uncertainty, I was inclined to wait, to hold off on what I communicated to the patients.

This response was motivated as well by a desire to protect myself and my patients. Although I was actively struggling to overcome a sense of helplessness and despair, the extent of my uncertainty was very difficult to tolerate. I assumed it would be hard for my patients to bear, not only because of their anxiety or fear, but also because they would be inactive, powerless bystanders. I didn't want to get involved in a running and shifting commentary on my circumstances. The turmoil any information could engender might be more than I wanted to, or would be able to, handle.

Self-preservation was the priority—in my pursuit of medical care, in directing my personal, emotional resources, and in protecting my privacy. I was therefore not prepared to explore the extent of my vulnerability or my terror and its impact on my patients. Nor was I particularly interested in delving into their feelings and fantasies about my unavailability. These impressions reinforced my wanting to say as little as possible.

On the other hand, inevitably, with many patients I had established (or was working to establish) an intimacy and a straightforwardness that made my refraining from being explicit feel absurd. The last-minute cancellations, the anxiety in my voice, could reveal a great deal, as could my frame of mind. I considered that I might not be around to speak with anyone three months hence. I felt this possibility could prompt an indiscriminate or uncontrolled candidness on my part, an illusory urgency, an impulse to communicate what I had previously failed to.

My situation affected my responsiveness at every moment. While this is nothing unusual, the extent and intensity of my preoccupation with my condition (independent of the patient) was unusually intrusive. Initially I wondered whether the intensified vulnerability might enhance my effectiveness as a therapist, although this notion struck me as compensatory and rationalizing.

The conventional form of a therapist's reserve, even in its modified contemporary version, felt like a shield, a piece of medieval armor. It left me estranged and dissociated. Continuing with business as usual involved too much dissembling.

So, very quickly, the structure of the therapeutic relationship broke down—in my mind, from my end. The options that presented themselves (my departure, precipitous leave, inability to affirm when and if I would return) collapsed the jointly held expectations about the collaborative therapeutic work. Whatever I chose to say or do would be disruptive and intrusive. There was no avoiding drawing considerable attention to myself. A burden would be placed on the patient, which, as the situation developed, would include his or her being cut off from normal channels of contact with me. While I tried to scrutinize my behavior and its impact, so many things were entirely out of my control. I worried that what I said or did might not be for the patient's benefit, would not be guided by the goal of advancing the therapeutic process. Personal anxiety gradually usurped my capacity to be attentive.[2]

In the first two weeks some patients chose not to ask much about the cancellations whereas others sharply questioned me. With each patient there were different steps in what I acknowledged and described, each step in part dependent on the fact that the situation was changing and what I knew at any given moment was in flux. Whatever the different steps, they were all taken within a very brief period, too short a time to titrate the information (as if that were possible or desirable) or to assess carefully what could be useful. From the outset, with most patients I openly conveyed what I knew. I granted a priority to the real situation, to that which we would hopefully live through together. There was insufficient time to unravel the impact of the knowledge of my illness on the patient and to gauge its meanings. Nor could we deal with the patient's compliance with what he or she imagined I wanted or the situation demanded.

During the very brief initial period when I answered only direct questions, a few patients experienced no cancellations (because of the time of day that I saw them), so our first relevant conversations had to do with the patient's queries about my responsiveness. One such patient, who knew nothing consciously about my illness but was someone whom I had previously experienced as sensing the nuances of my more internal emotional states, asserted, following a remark of mine that had disturbed him, "Something is wrong with you.

Something is definitely wrong!" Under other circumstances I might have found this remark disturbing or funny (taking it as a given) and been curious, possibly played with it. Here, however, I simply assented internally and presented a mournful affect. My lack of a more engaged response contributed to what immediately followed: the patient stormed out of my office.

Another patient, Mark, had spoken for several months about his upcoming wedding, an event of immense significance in his life. Among the many aspects Mark grappled with in our work was that his father had said he would not be coming to the wedding because of a prior engagement. The father's anger, often simmering, had been inflamed owing to circumstances to which Mark had indirectly contributed. Specifically, the father had found out about the wedding date from someone other than his son.

Mark's characteristic distancing behavior generally protected him from his father's wrath and limited Mark's own sadness, anger, and pain. Yet it could also, as in this instance, elicit the father's fury. When this happened, Mark's detachment turned the tables on his father, so that his father felt *he* was repudiated, treated like an unrelated, impotent entity. Mark's father, never acknowledging he was hurt and bitter, maintained for several months that he would not be coming simply because of another obligation. At the very last moment, however, he decided to attend.

The wedding ceremony was scheduled for September 25th, which was at the end of the week when I informed patients that I would be taking a medical leave. I had decided that I would not say anything about my illness to Mark prior to his wedding; I assumed I could inform him the following week. At the last session before his wedding, however, Mark told me he was going on a honeymoon and would be away for several weeks. There had been no reason to believe he was leaving, and I was thus faced with the likelihood that I would not be able to inform him in person or speak with him before I took the medical leave (or possibly, ever again).

I was momentarily furious (like his father, perhaps) at Mark's neglecting to let me know about his plans. Similar things had occurred in our past together and had sometimes been shocking: Mark's fogginess or forgetfulness, his disavowal of intention, his apparent lack of consideration. Yet the intensity of my present response was very much colored and deepened by my unacknowledged condition.

Mark had invited me to the ceremony and I had thought I would attend. But my fury at his behavior entered into my decision not to go. Coming also into play was that on the particular weekend in question I did not want to take any additional time away from being with my wife and children. Nor did I want to be alone for the several hours of driving that attendance at the ceremony would require. I might not have gone solely for these reasons. However, the turn of events transformed Mark's "neglect" of me into something quite painful: it intensified my feeling of being cut off, shut out, mishandled, fiercely disconnected (feelings which were familiar states to Mark and to our work, although generally much more muted). While Mark's failure to imagine and perceive the impact of his actions was something I had previously experienced, I had never before felt it so deeply. I did recognize, though, that what I felt corresponded to some of the patient's experience as a child, when he was on the receiving end of immensely isolating and hurtful behavior.

Is That Your Tumor Talking?

On September 20th, 11 days after I learned of my tumor, I began to inform my patients that I would be taking a medical leave, beginning in two weeks. This decision followed informal discussion with colleagues and within my personal analysis. Based on what I knew at that point, I told my patients I would be away from work for at least two months. I said I expected that I would be contacting them by the end of October with more specific information about when I would be returning to work. There was evident uncertainty, and those patients who didn't know quickly surmised or were informed that I was facing a life-threatening illness. All my patients asked for some details and I told them what I knew. In most cases we met for about two weeks after the overt disclosure. Following that, I tried to preserve some structure, through covering therapists and optional referrals, which I hoped would permit resuming work at some point. I also tried to keep open a channel of communication by telling patients they could speak with the covering therapists, who would be apprised of my medical situation.

On certain days and with some patients, I am sure my intense vulnerability and terror were particularly evident. Once the issue had been opened with a patient, he or she regularly asked about my circumstances and thus drew us into a conversation that I dreaded (and at times sought). In regard to this, I was mildly concerned that I might be relying on my patients, depending on them (for support, encouragement, and care) in ways that might not be in their interest. I also thought I could no longer evaluate any of this. But I operated with a basic conviction that, given the life-and-death situation, the imposing reality of what I, and we, were facing, talking with the patients about the circumstances, including aspects of my experience, would inevitably be of value. That may have been self-serving, but under the circumstances, serving myself emotionally seemed inevitable and defensible. Yet the tables didn't turn entirely (or even mostly). In some sessions, for about 20 minutes, overt focus might be on my predicament and the uncertainty of our situation, but invariably it returned to the patient and his or her experience (and this was frequently a relief).

It was during the two-week interim that many patients expressed their fear that I might die, and most conveyed their love and support. One patient suggested that I was growing an extra brain in order to help her more effectively.

Another patient responded to what seemed like a particularly outlandish remark of mine (I had made some reference to the cow in formaldehyde that was then being exhibited at the Brooklyn Museum) by saying, "Is that your tumor talking?" This patient's question wryly acknowledged the presence of my illness in the room, its palpable silence, and her uncertainty about it, her ongoing effort to detect its influence. I had to admit she was on to something. The tumor was behind my eyes at all times and yet it was sightless and invisible; it didn't literally blur my vision although it skewed it. It was beneath my brain, on its edge, but it was senseless. It prompted lots of talk, yet it had been totally, distressingly inarticulate.

There came a point—the last week that I worked—when I simply felt I could not continue. I had envisioned arriving at this juncture. I stopped six weeks before my treatment began and well before I even knew what it would be. But the fact was I could no longer concentrate or focus enough on my patients and on what was going on between us. There were extended moments in which my looking to some patients for understanding came to the foreground. I was too anxious and preoccupied, and the responsibility to sort things out was more than I could bear.

Higher Court Ruling

On Tuesday, September 28th, at around noon (and only 19 days after the sun had disappeared behind the clouds), I called Dr. Bloch at Beth Israel. He was covering for Dr. Logan and he returned my call later in the afternoon. He told me that he had contacted the pathology lab at Sloan-Kettering (I had left him the phone number and asked him to do so); he had tried to find out what was happening with my biopsy tissue. Dr. Bloch informed me that he had been told that the original diagnosis, an adenocarcinoma, had now been ruled out. He said they were pursuing the possibility that the mass was a low-grade neuroendocrine tumor, possibly an esthesioneuroblastoma or a pituitary gland tumor. Dr. Bloch said he had made some suggestions to the pathologists for avenues to pursue. He said that they were having a hard time pinning the tumor down, identifying the type and source, that it seemed exceedingly rare. He told me this raised anew the question of surgery; everything was again up in the air. He noted that it was definitely good news—the types of cancer being considered were less invasive, less infiltrative, relatively more benign. He made sure to emphasize, "This is good news."

I was ecstatic. I let out a tremendous sigh of relief. I had been given a reprieve. My death sentence was temporarily commuted. I was cautious, but I clearly heard that I was better off. My good fortune, arbitrary as it was, felt exhilarating. I recalled George's warnings that good news could readily be followed by bad (and when I spoke with him he was sure to remind me of this fact). But I was delighted, though still feeling hurled about by something very much out of my control and having no apparent relation to me. I called Suzie, other members of my family, and my friend Eric. I cried intensely, as did several of those I spoke with.

The following day I called the Sloan-Kettering doctors, Samuel, Hughes, and Barnet (who had been away), but was unable to reach any of them.

Two days later, on Thursday, September 30th, I met with Dr. Samuel, the medical oncologist at Sloan-Kettering. He explained to me that he had been on call at the hospital for his annual two-week stint, and this was why it had been so difficult to reach him and schedule an appointment. He mentioned that he ordinarily saw patients in a different space but was seeing me in that particular office because he was still on call and had to squeeze me in. He told me, matter-of-factly and without comment, that he had received phone calls from several of my friends who were doctors.

Dr. Samuel had been billed as *the* expert in the world on head tumors and chemotherapy. Dr. Logan at Beth Israel had said Samuel was the best, had the widest knowledge base and experience, and related very well to his patients. Logan had even speculated that I might want to split my treatment between Samuel at Sloan-Kettering for chemotherapy and Dr. Rief at Beth Israel for radiation.

A short, graying man in his 60s, Dr. Samuel did not know that the pathology lab at his own hospital had changed the diagnosis. I initially assumed he knew, but when I realized he wasn't aware, I quickly informed him. Samuel then said (and repeated several times subsequently) that he had anticipated a straightforward consultation, but now things were quite uncertain. Dr. Samuel had a habit of thinking out loud and repeating himself, so much so that at moments he seemed to be almost perseverative. He would return over and over again to the same thought without any shift or addition. I tolerated this silently, assuming it was a habit of thought and hoping, at each go-round, that something new would emerge.

He called the pathology lab and basically repeated to me what Dr. Bloch from Beth Israel had said two days earlier. Apparently five or six people were working on the pathology slides and they were still not prepared to "sign out" the results. This meant that there was more uncertainty than they found acceptable, and they continued to try to narrow down the possibilities. Dr. Samuel also indicated that the surgical option might now be reconsidered. He said he would speak with colleagues because of the rarity of the tumor. Despite his vast experience, he had not seen one like it in terms of pathology, location, and size. He wondered if it might "ring a bell" with someone else. He thought it made sense to speak with doctors around the country. He said the tumor would present certain technical difficulties for surgery, but perhaps someone had developed means for dealing with these difficulties. He called in his colleague Dr. Hughes because he wanted to view the MRI that had been left in her possession, and she came to the latter half of the consultation. She too said she would consult with colleagues around the country via e-mail to see if anyone had experience with a tumor of this type. While the news was good that the initial diagnosis was wrong, it became apparent that the difficulty in identifying the tumor, its extreme rarity, presented considerable problems for treatment.

The lower court ruling had not been completely vacated.

Two Very Different Kinds of People

The following evening, Friday, October 1st, Dr. Barnet called me at home. I carried our portable phone into a room out of range of our children and, pacing back and forth, strained to be attentive. He told me he had consulted extensively at Sloan-Kettering and "with five or six colleagues around the country." He said that Sloan-Kettering had reached an "institutional decision" regarding how to proceed.

I understood those two words, uttered authoritatively, as indicating, at a minimum, that Dr. Barnet had spoken with the other doctors involved in my case, Dr. Samuel and Dr. Hughes. I assumed that he probably had also spoken with other physicians at the hospital and that there was a consensus about the treatment recommendations he was about to tell me.

Dr. Barnet reported that, despite the change in the tumor's pathology, surgical resection was still out of the question. He noted that the recommendation against craniofacial surgery in such an instance was the subject of a talk he had just given at some conference outside the country. The new recommendation was for a partial endoscopic resection: an attempt would be made to remove as much of the tumor as possible, endoscopically, through the nose. Dr. Barnet said he would perform the surgery using a machine called a "brain lab," and that this aspect of the procedure would involve the participation of a neurosurgeon. Barnet thought he could remove about 80% of the tumor this way. I asked a couple of questions but felt I needed some time to consider things; I therefore indicated I would like to meet with him to discuss the new recommendation. He sounded surprised at my request but was obliging and arranged for an appointment the following Monday.

At first the recommendation seemed to be something of a compromise, an apparently less risky but still aggressive approach. Being a compromise, it was appealing to both Suzie and me, and we laughed at our common perception. We were relieved that the prospective dangerous surgery might be avoided. One of my physician-friends said that she too found it attractive as a middle road, but then qualified this sentiment by acknowledging that it was only a temperamental preference. I remained quite unclear about the benefit of such surgery.

When we saw Dr. Barnet on Monday he made a verbal gesture indicating that, as I was the last patient of the day, we would have as much time as needed to discuss my concerns. I began by asking what I took to be simple layman's questions based on common sense. I asked about the benefits of a partial resection, to which Barnet responded that the benefit of the "debulking" was the help it would provide to the radiation. He indicated that it would permit a redistribution of the radiation, making it possible to increase the amount to some areas because of the reduction in size of the tumor.

I tried to have him clarify why this would be so, but Dr. Barnet quickly became impatient. He evidently felt that I was asking too many questions, doubting his authority. He said, "David, *you and I are two very different kinds of people!* . . . If I have a problem I simply go to the best guy to fix it. When I'm faced with a decision, I get the expert and that's it. If something needs to be done at my house, I tell my wife: Find the best. Period!"

The implication was clear: he wanted me to share in the assumption that he was the best. He should not have to bother with maintaining my trust. Dr. Barnet seemed to be impatient with my uncertainty about the proposed surgery, with my seeking commonsense clarification, and he sought to bisect our common humanity, to separate himself from me, to place us in opposing categories. It is my retrospective interpretation that his behavior was motivated by an impulse *to* identify with me which he could not tolerate. Perhaps it also arose from some residual anxiety about his clinical choice and its rationale, including the manner in which he had presented them to me.

I was upset, disappointed, and angry. I muttered something along the lines that I was not redecorating my house. Yet it was exceedingly difficult to contend with Dr. Barnet's assertion of authority, beneath which lay the authority of his institution. I was still not inclined to dismiss Dr. Barnet, despite his behavior. I had in mind the person who had recommended him (Dr. Mills) and the generic folk wisdom with regard to surgeons. When the appointment was over, I scheduled the suggested surgery, the partial resection, for Friday of the following week (October 15th). This also meant scheduling preoperative testing, a preparatory encounter with "brain lab," an MRI, and canceling the radiation.

While I did have an impulse to accept Dr. Barnet's authority, I also wanted to check, to confirm it with others, to have it constructed within my hearing and before my eyes. In the days following, on my own initiative, I called Dr. Barnet's colleagues at Sloan-Kettering. Dr. Samuel, the medical oncologist, expressed surprise when told of Barnet's recommendation and said he was not at all aware of what Barnet had referred to as an "institutional decision." With characteristic restraint, he said, "This is not a one-man show, but a multimodal approach." He said he wanted to perform other tests before the proposed surgery, tests whose results might affect the schedule and sequence of treatments and delay the surgery. For example, he wanted me to have an octreotide scan to test for the tumor's receptiveness to certain radioactive isotopes. Samuel reiterated that there was no known treatment for this tumor because of its rarity; there was no protocol, no scientific evidence in support of a particular course of chemotherapy.

Nothing Palliative

I continued to speak with all my friends, with whom I reviewed the consultations and other information. I remember distinctly only a few of these conversations. One was at a dinner we had with neighbors, both of whom are doctors at prestigious institutions: Ina, a gynecologist, and Ira, an endocrinologist and researcher. On a few occasions I had asked them to help me with research on the Internet—for example, into the type of tumor I had and potential treatments and outcomes. That evening Ira presented me with a small sheaf of papers, six or eight abstracts on neuroendocrine tumors and octreotide agents. I gathered from his impressions and a cursory glance at the limited research and literature that very little was known about how to treat low-grade neuroendocrine tumors in the head. Whatever significant literature there was pertained to neuro-endocrine tumors elsewhere in the body. The information on octreotides was scant, experimental, and inconclusive. It was clear that, in mentioning the possibility of octreotide treatment, Dr. Samuel (along with Dr. Satlovski, who had also brought up this option) was reaching quite a bit in re-sponse to a rare tumor for which no experimentally tested treatments existed.

The discussion over dinner that evening turned on two other matters as well. Ira said he was convinced that treat-ment of cancer, based on recent biological research and the general advancement of medicine, would be transformed within the next five years. New treatments would be devel-oped that might genuinely revolutionize cancer care. This claim has repeatedly been made at various times over the past 20 years, but Ira felt that developments in molecular bi-ology offered firm hope that cancer would soon be treated very differently. Yet what conclusion to draw from this as far as my situation was concerned was unclear. For exam-ple, did this mean I should not take too grave a risk in the present; if I could survive for a few years, more benign and effective treatments might well be available. Ira tried to communicate a general hopefulness, an attitude that, if all else fails now, other possibilities may come along soon.

In a different and seemingly contradictory vein, he noted that I was young and should not settle for a non-aggressive treatment, for something palliative, for a treat-ment that didn't aim at cure. He and Ina argued strongly for pursuing the surgical option as far as possible. In this con-text Ina brought up the name of a very prominent neuro-surgeon at Mount Sinai, Dr. Crowley, a name that had been mentioned by other sources. I had already begun a consultation process at Sinai with Dr. Satlovski, and, language comprehension troubles notwithstanding, had provided them with a good set of films and a slide for their pathologist to review. I had not yet met with the surgical part of their Head and Neck Oncology Department, but, with Ina's encouragement, I now decided to do so.

Other conversations that I had, some with my brother-in-law, Joe, also left me with the feeling I should consult further. Several people mentioned hospitals elsewhere in the country, including M. D. Anderson in Texas and the Mayo Clinic, and encouraged me to consider them. I had the idea that I would pursue what was available in New York first, and therefore made appointments with Dr. Crowley at Sinai and Dr. Martin, a neurosurgeon at Columbia. Several different people had recommended Martin. One source of referral, a neurologist who worked at the same hospital and a friend of a friend, had been full of praise for him; another source had described him as trying to establish his reputation and therefore perhaps inclined to take risks that others would not. I thought it was worth a visit, although I knew he would perform the surgery with Dr. Scheuer, the ENT with whom I already had had one memorable encounter.

A Shadow of Opportunity

*O*n the 28th day, in the second month, Suzie and I met with Dr. Martin. He was a well-known neurosurgeon and, if you're keeping score, the eighth doctor I had consulted. So far there had been one ENT specialist, three ENT oncology surgeons, one radiation oncologist, and two medical oncologists. This tally, which was still ascending, is for actuarial purposes only.

Dr. Martin was the usual hour and a half late. When we were told he was ready to see us, we were ushered into a large room with an impressive view, a mammoth desk, and lots of fine wood furniture. As we waited further, we played our game, encouraging Dr. Martin to come out of hiding, and I wondered aloud if my vision had now been affected as I couldn't see the doctor we had been told was awaiting us.

When he finally made his entrance, Dr. Martin, a handsome man in his 50s, appeared confident and relatively comfortable. His style was direct and clear, and he was patient in answering all our questions. The consultation lasted about an hour and a half, and I called a few days later to ask several additional questions.

Martin said that the majority of the surgeries that he performed, about 200 a year, were within the brain—some with considerably higher risks than there would be with my tumor. In my case Martin strongly advocated surgery, arguing that we had a "window of opportunity" (to my ears, a Vietnam War era phrase) which would be available for perhaps only a few months. In other words, if the tumor grew a bit more, surgery would definitely be out of the question. As it was, it would be risky but manageable. The window-of-opportunity argument involved further discussion of the sequence of different treatments. If chemotherapy was first, in an effort to shrink the tumor and thus make it potentially more amenable to surgery, it would delay surgery, and if it failed, perhaps foreclose the possibility altogether. Chemotherapy itself might damage the surrounding healthy tissue, thus requiring us to wait before proceeding with other treatment. Inversely, if surgery preceded chemotherapy and it failed, it could cause considerable, irreparable damage and, because of the resultant inflammation and scar tissue, make the assessment of the effects of chemotherapy difficult if not impossible. As radiation also damages tissue, healthy and cancerous alike, similar considerations pertained to its position in a sequence of treatments. I felt like a child in a toy store.

While reviewing the films, Martin showed how they were inconclusive as to whether the tumor had broken into the cavernous sinus, that highly sensitive passageway containing the carotid artery carrying blood to the brain. Nonetheless he believed he might be able to remove 90% to 100% of the tumor. He outlined the risks. The primary one was to my vision. There was also a risk of irreversible stroke and paralysis, due to the proximity of the tumor to the carotid artery. There was a risk of short-term memory loss, of my balance and gait being temporarily affected, as well as impairment of my "higher cognitive functions" owing to the frontal-lobe manipulation. These last few would likely be temporary side effects, like those from a concussion. There was also a risk of spinal fluid leakage, but this was slight. And there were the general risks associated with anesthesia and surgery. While Dr. Martin assessed the risk of any one of the complications as between 1% and 5%, he thought the likelihood of one of the complications occurring was between 5% and 10%. Dr. Martin also indicated he would like a neuropathologist at his hospital to look at my biopsy slides. I subsequently arranged for this and the pathologist concurred with the diagnosis of the pathologists at Memorial.

The principal issue around the surgery, then, had to do with the risk–benefit ratio. In understanding the benefit, focus was on how much tumor could be safely removed. If the tumor could not be removed in its entirety, and 1% to 2% or 5% to 20% remained, what was the benefit, given that malignant cells were left behind, some in the most dangerous, vulnerable areas, and these cells would continue to grow in any of the possible directions? As Suzie and I moved through the various consultations, we received different answers to this question—obviously some doctors believed

that removing 90% to 95% of the tumor would be benefi-
cial, while others thought that this wouldn't accomplish
much, and that the percentage of removed tumor had to be
significantly higher. As one would expect, radiation oncologists seemed to think surgery would be less effective than
the surgeons thought. Several surgeons appeared to believe
that, once the tumor was removed, the field of radiation
would be smaller and the radiation more focused. But the
radiation oncologists insisted that, following surgery, the
entire initial volume of the tumor would need to be irradi-
ated because there would be uncertainty about whether or
not microscopic cancerous cells had been left behind. In
addition, if the entire tumor could not be extracted, surgery
could result in scar tissue or damage to the tumor's blood
supply, both of which might reduce the effectiveness of radiation. I formed the impression, based on the various discussions, that surgery would be worth the risk only if close
to 100% of the tumor could be removed.

Despite some awkwardness, I raised several touchy
questions with Dr. Martin. I first asked about his collaboration with Dr. Scheuer, the ENT surgeon. I mentioned
some aspects of my experience with Scheuer, particularly
the issue of whether or not a biopsy was called for. Martin's
response showed that he was already aware of my reservations about Dr. Scheuer, probably from colleagues of
friends of mine who worked at the hospital. He said he
would perform about 70% of the surgery, and Dr. Scheuer
would do 30%. He expressed respect for Dr. Scheuer and
defended some aspects of the latter's reservations about
the necessity of a biopsy, although he carefully indicated
that he thought a biopsy had been appropriate. In response to another question, Dr. Martin said, with some

slight hesitation, that he would still have recommended surgery even if the diagnosis had remained adenocarcinoma. When I asked what he thought about a partial resection done endoscopically (Dr. Barnet's plan), Martin appeared to dismiss its value and conveyed the clear sense that it offered no benefit whatsoever.

At one point I asked Dr. Martin who the medical and radiation oncologists on his team would be, and he replied vaguely, saying there were several possibilities. Evidently he felt this was not the time to mention any names. His thinking may have been that, if I chose him to be the surgeon, the choice of other specialists could be worked out later. While that may have been true, it didn't leave me with the feeling that a team would be functioning from the outset with the full advantage of different perspectives and kinds of expertise.

Somewhere during the course of the interview, Suzie referred to the photographs on Dr. Martin's desk and asked him about his children in an unsuccessful effort to reduce some of the rigid formality of the proceedings. But Martin would not shift his demeanor to establish a different kind of personal connection.

I also asked Dr. Martin whom he would consult with outside New York were he in my position. He appeared put off by the question and visibly stiffened in response: "Oh, there are several major medical centers outside the city." His nonanswer and his manner conveyed to me that he thought the question inappropriate, even illegitimate. He was obviously not going to recommend a particular place or individual.

Nonetheless, Suzie and I left the meeting buoyed by the possibility of a successful treatment. This was despite the fact that I thought it unlikely that I would proceed with surgery performed by Dr. Martin. He appeared bright, thorough, controlled, and confident, but the depth of his confidence was not convincing, and his arguments left me quite uncertain as to the value of what he could do.

The window of opportunity was more a barely perceptible shadow, like some of the critical fragments in the images on the scans.

Contradiction

That same afternoon I spoke again with Dr. Logan at Beth Israel to ascertain his hospital's final recommendations. In a measured and somber tone, Logan reported that his team had concluded that, despite the change in diagnosis, surgery would still be too risky. Consequently, they were proposing chemotherapy and radiation, to run concurrently. When I told him that Dr. Samuel at Sloan-Kettering, whom Logan had previously acknowledged to be preeminent in his field, had indicated that there was no obvious protocol for chemotherapy, Dr. Logan deferred to his judgment: "Well, if that's what Dr. Samuel says." His tone was sad, even mournful, as though he knew he wasn't offering much.

I asked Logan about the notion of a partial resection done endoscopically. He seemed to scoff at the idea. He said an 80% tumor removal, a so-called debulking, would be of no benefit and carried considerable risk. He said there would be little way to know how close the surgeon was coming to vital structures, and one drop of blood could appear like a flood on the screen. Logan noted that, although the pathologists had identified the tumor as low-grade, "it is not behaving like a low-grade tumor." By this he was referring to the fact that the tumor appeared to have destroyed a lot of tissue and bone. Logan concluded our discussion with the sobering, "I am sorry that you have to go through this. . . . God bless you."

Although the team at Beth Israel appeared to be offering relatively little hope, the next day I made an appointment with Dr. Rief, the radiation oncologist at that hospital, as he had been recommended as the best in *his* field. While hesitant and weary, I chose to be persistent and aimed for the goal of greater comprehensiveness.

That evening Suzie and I were both filled with extraordinary tension. In a handful of hours we had received two antithetical opinions (Martin's and Logan's, Columbia's and Beth Israel's) about how to proceed, neither of which felt particularly optimistic or assured. As far as we could tell, the third opinion (Sloan-Kettering's) was not internally coherent; it was not consistent with either of the other two recommendations and had received no external support. Was clarity or consensus even a possibility? Was I running out of time?

As Suzie and I continued our rounds, I said more than once, "I don't know how long I can keep this up. I think we need to decide on a treatment course soon . . . perhaps by the end of next week, latest." And then another week would go by and I would say the same thing. Suzie would nod and she would hold me.

Stuffed Animal

Twenty-nine days after I first learned of my tumor was the last day I saw my patients. The leave taking was provisional. I arranged for five different colleagues to cover specific patients and to be available by phone or in person if the patient chose. (Only one patient, someone who had recently begun working with me, elected to be referred permanently to another therapist.) I said I would not be available by phone because I could not guarantee I would be able to return calls in a timely fashion. I told my patients I would contact them within a month to let them know what my plans were and when I would be able to return to work. Many patients expressed their gratitude to me, their affection, and their concern. Some of these statements were made with an explicit background of "if we don't see each other again."

At our last session, Ellen, a 27-year-old woman working for a large Wall Street firm, gave me a beloved object from her childhood, a stuffed dog, to keep temporarily. An implication was that if I held on to the dog it would protect me. I accepted this gift with thanks, but in an awkward, embarrassed fashion that reflected my ambivalence. The patient mentioned that the dog was one of several, a means conceived by her mother for protecting against wear and tear and loss. Ellen noted that her mother had fooled her in order to wash the stuffed dog, and Ellen had been astonished to learn this as an adult. She warned me, in a jocular fashion, against losing the stuffed animal; she had formerly had five but had given one to a friend making a trip who was afraid of traveling on her own, and the friend had lost it.

Ellen pointed out certain features of the dog she was giving me: its worn fur, a torn ear. She described how the animal got so much use when she was a child that it came to lose its facial features.

My feelings in accepting the dog involved a recognition of Ellen's desire to remain in touch and to be giving. But they also entailed a reaction to her warning that I had to care for the animal (which I didn't want to) and return it safely (which I wasn't sure I could). Her cautions meant that this wasn't simply a gift for me to use as I wished. It felt more like a responsibility—and one I was not sure I could fulfill. Another feeling was my dismissal of a desire for such an object, the feeling that there was no available magical protection, none I wanted to rely on or could resort to. I was also uncomfortable with what Ellen had described as her mother's deception, which I imagined I might be perpetrating in some analogous way by taking the dog into my care.

Ellen's mother's behavior was intended to prevent the patient's experiencing absence or loss for even a moment, feelings that unfortunately were quite present in the child's life. In particular, her father's attachment to Ellen and her mother was miserably unreliable, even fraudulent. The stuffed animal deception was of a piece with other parental behaviors that staved off the patient's awareness of her father's cruel unavailability. They blocked any process within the patient that would have permitted a gradual disillusionment regarding her father; instead, the feeling was fostered that she had to win and hold on to him at all costs. Ellen was mystified as to what constituted a reliable and desirable object.

I left the stuffed dog in a drawer of a cabinet in my office. I felt that in some measure I was deceiving Ellen, fooling her, pretending that the care I would bestow on the stuffed animal would be continuous and genuine, pretending that I wanted to hold on to the object or to her. At the time, I was not open to the stuffed dog as a symbol of our attachment and its survival. Nor could I fully face the rending of our relationship and its possible dissolution by my death. In that moment, in that context, I took the dog much too concretely. I did not want to pretend anything.

Another patient, Ben, responded to the circumstances of our parting with anxiety and fear. A 28-year-old man who writes fiction and was a doctoral student in literature, Ben had entered therapy in a state of panic and desperation. In the preceding six weeks he had had severe sleep difficulties, and when we first met he had been almost entirely unable to sleep for over a week. These difficulties were palpably related to Ben's fears of being alone and separate. He had experienced similar problems for a period in his childhood when he could fall asleep only in close proximity to his brother. Shortly after we began working together, I referred him for medication, which, along with the therapy, helped to moderate his symptoms. In the course of the year and a half we worked together prior to my illness, Ben had gone off the medication without having a recurrence of the severe sleeplessness. When I told him of my medical leave, however, he was terrified. Only much later did he tell me that he had been scared he would collapse and experience a devastating regression.

In the last two sessions before my medical leave, Ben posed several questions concerning his loyalty to me. He was at first reluctant to express these sentiments, but his resistance was relatively slight, and his subsequent remarks were conveyed emphatically and with relief. He wondered what would happen if he became attached to the therapist covering for me and even came to prefer that person. The reasons for the imagined preference remained obscure but overtly had to do with the patient's desire for a therapist who would more quickly and capably resolve his sleep difficulties. Beneath this question appeared an edge of hostility, the sense that "if you're going to leave me, I might as well abandon you first."

These thoughts aroused in Ben feelings of embarrassment and guilt. At the time I was initially affected by what felt like callousness on his part. His manner of speculating on the possibilities appeared strikingly aloof, with an aspect of innocence and disregard of our intimacy and attachment. However, this was not deliberate or conscious, but rather an expression of Ben's inability to tolerate the feelings of loss. His thoughts seemed to protect him from feeling too dependent and from being overwhelmed by fear at the severing of our attachment. Although I was hurt and pained by his considerations, I didn't say so. I was embedded with him in the traumatic atmosphere, and we did not have time to discuss his terror, my terror, his overt detachment, my disengagement, and the intensity of our involvement and affection.

In response to another patient, Margaret, who inquired about my children in our last session, I showed her some photographs of them. Moments later this gesture struck me as primarily having to do with my personal preoccupation. I was looking to the patient to care for me in a way I almost immediately found troublesome. Although I subsequently thought about why I had chosen to exhibit to this patient my parental attachment and to display my anxiety and pride, I remained uneasy about my action. I cannot say, though, that it negatively affected our work together. Rather, it actually seemed to promote the patient's development toward an easing of our separation and a greater comfort with her own maternal feelings.

A fourth patient, Roland, offered me very tangible help. On my last day at work, he mentioned that he had a childhood friend (now in his mid 50s), practically a family member, who was currently a chief of neurosurgery in Tel Aviv. He asked if I wanted him to contact Dr. Ouaknine for me. As I was pursuing almost every possibility and thought someone from outside New York or the United States might have a valuable suggestion, I said, "Sure, go ahead." I said this despite obvious reservations about accepting such an offer of help from a patient.

New York, New York

*O*n the evening of the 29th day (October 8th), I received a return call from Dr. Hughes, the radiation oncologist at Sloan-Kettering. When I described to her Dr. Barnet's plan, she, like Dr. Samuel, was surprised. In addition, when I raised a question concerning Dr. Barnet's expressed reason for the partial resection—that it would enable the radiation to be distributed differently—she flatly stated, "Dr. Barnet doesn't understand radiation." Thus two of the three physicians on the Memorial team appeared unaware of the "institutional decision" and did not necessarily agree with it.

Hughes noted that there was an unproven clinical sense that the same amount of radiation directed in the same manner could work better on a smaller piece of tumor, although this had not been scientifically demonstrated. However, the suggested resection evidently meant nothing in terms of diminishing or redistributing the amount of radiation to be used. Dr. Hughes conveyed that she had discussed my case with both a former teacher and a supervisor, two people she often consulted with. They had concurred with her plan, which was to direct a moderate dose to include the entire tumor volume and a high-tech boost to the cavernous sinus.

At one point toward the end of our conversation, Hughes said, with a tone of natural curiosity and only a little exasperation, "Is this all you think about? Why don't you take a break, put it aside, let *us* worry about it?" But then, before I could respond, she said, "What am I saying? You're a psychotherapist." She then wished me a peaceful weekend.

I was dumbfounded at Dr. Barnet's apparent failure to communicate with his colleagues. He had laid claim to institutional authority for a decision about which the other doctors involved in my case had no knowledge. He seemed to expect deference and appeared not to anticipate that I would want access to the decision-making process or that I would speak with the other physicians. In subsequent consultations at other institutions, I broached Barnet's suggestion of endoscopic surgery and received uniformly negative judgments: it was thought to be both too risky and of no demonstrable benefit.

Thus, after speaking with Samuel and Hughes, I canceled the preoperative testing, the encounter with "brain lab," and the surgery, and scheduled the octreotide scan for the following week. I would be injected with a radioisotope and then monitored twice, 4 hours later and 24 hours later, to see if the tumor took up the isotope, thereby indicating it might shrink in response to a treatment with the octreotide agent.

The next day, my patient Roland left a message on my answering machine at work. He had spoken with his childhood friend in Israel. If I wanted to call, Dr. Ouaknine would be available in his office the next day, between 3 A.M. and 5 A.M. New York time. That night, before going to sleep, feeling exhausted and wondering whether there was any point in following this lead, I put my radiology and pathology reports out on the table beside the phone and set the alarm for 3 A.M. I thought this might be foolhardy, excessive, adding yet another cook to spoil a broth that was already unsavory and indigestible. I went to sleep still doubting I would make the call.

Hours later Dr. Ouaknine quickly came to the phone. I began to read him the reports, but after the first three lines or so, getting the gist, conveying impatience in a clipped and rapid manner, and with a French and Israeli accent, he said, "This must come out. There are three doctors in the U.S. I would recommend. I will fax their phone numbers and addresses." The doctors he referred to were Dr. Espinal in Pittsburgh, Dr. Gallagher in Washington, DC, and Dr. Neria in Boston.

Dr. Neria's name had been mentioned to me already in another context. My sister Leslie had a friend in Boston, Denise, who, on learning of my illness, had begun researching among doctors in Boston to find out who would be the best ones to consult. (So had my brother-in-law and other friends who had contacts in Boston; however, they either came up with other names or no one at all.) Denise e-mailed Leslie almost daily, so it seemed. Each time she came up with a variety of new names and a host of suggestions. Leslie would pass on the e-mails to me. The notes were telegraphic and high-pitched, scurrying about among different leads. They appeared inconsistent, even incoherent, and for these reasons I only skimmed them, giving a cursory glance to their contents, thereby adding to my sense of their disorder. Reading them was dizzying: go here; no, go there; this one's the best; no, this one; call and say this. The notes were bursting with what appeared to be impractical and contradictory advice about how to proceed with establishing contact and providing for a reasonable consultation. I couldn't help but believe that whoever Denise spoke with would receive only very partial and perhaps inaccurate information as to my situation. I was also aware that my sister's friend had had more than her share of ailments, some of which were debilitating. I had heard that she had seen a multitude of doctors and healers.

I did learn, however, that prior to changing professions and becoming disabled, Denise had been an oncology nurse. It was also the case that amid all the noise and clutter, one of Denise's e-mails, dated September 23rd, concluded that, based on several referral sources, the person I should see was Dr. Neria. Denise described him as the head of a consortium of doctors from all the Boston hospitals and all the specialties that focused on treating tumors in the base of the skull.

I have copies of the e-mails and have read them many times since. Each time I do, I am deeply moved by Denise's activity on my behalf. We had met only briefly, two or three times. But in her e-mails, Denise seemed capable of intensely identifying with the terror and vulnerability of my situation. Perhaps that's why she made so many phone calls and spoke extensively with several people. Her notes now appear far more coherent and intelligible than my initial reading led me to believe.

Until this point I had refrained from actively pursuing specific options outside the city. I first wanted to clarify the diagnosis and the recommendations I was receiving in New York. Manhattan alone had many reputable institutions with renowned doctors, and I was consulting at four of them. But I was coming to the belated conclusion that Manhattan was insular. In a way it had never appeared to me before, it felt claustrophobic, with doctors jockeying for position and prestige.

At about this time, Suzie received a message at work that someone affiliated with her school had been trying to reach her. It turned out that this person was related to someone high up in the administration of Memorial Sloan-Kettering. She wanted to offer any help she could, especially as she had heard we were having some difficulties with the institution. Very soon thereafter, Lydia, from the senior administrator's office, contacted us. It appeared that she was in charge of patient relations, and she offered us her help. She had been led to believe that our problem was primarily a difference of opinion between Memorial and other hospitals. While I was concerned about navigating things diplomatically, I felt directness was preferable. I simply indicated that, yes, there were differing opinions but a significant problem at Sloan-Kettering was that the team was not functioning as a team; the doctors were not communicating with one another. Surprised and hinting that such a matter might well be outside her purview, Lydia said she would see what she could do.

My phone call with Dr. Ouaknine, halfway around the world, led me to make a move. Thirty-two days after Dr.

Gibson helped me to make a 10-dollar investment in a future eventuality, I called Dr. Neria's office in Boston. I left a message describing the size, location, and pathology of the tumor. Dr. Neria returned my call in a few hours and suggested that I FedEx him the CT scan and MRI along with the reports. I did this the following day.

Hopes and Prayers

Mildly queasy after 33 days on the roiling seas, Suzie and I sailed into the offices of Dr. Crowley, a leading neurosurgeon at Mount Sinai. He had been recommended by several friends who thought surgery in the base of the skull was his specialty. Seeing him would also extend the consultation process at Sinai, where I had already met with Dr. Satlovski, the medical oncologist. Immediately upon being introduced to Dr. Crowley, however, he brought us to see Dr. Blair, who Crowley said was the surgical specialist in the relevant anatomical region.

As was the case in our other consultations, Dr. Blair began by reviewing the films. Close to the outset of the interview, when Blair was conveying some optimism about the possibility for surgery, Suzie asked, "So our boys won't lose their father?" To which Dr. Blair responded, "No, I don't think so."

Yet, as his perusal of the scans continued, he increasingly emphasized the risks and limitations of surgery. He noted that the tumor had broken into the clivus (the bone separating the sinus cavities from the brain stem, and a specific anatomical part we had yet to hear referred to by this name). He thought the tumor itself might be plugging the hole it had created through its own destructive expansion, and any effort to remove the tumor there could lead to spinal fluid leakage. This potential leakage could range from something quite manageable to something that would be very difficult to stop and could result in death within a relatively short time period. The problem might necessitate a difficult reconstruction of the bone during the process of the surgery.

Dr. Blair did say, "People don't die on the table anymore." And, "It's been years since I lost a patient under similar circumstances." These remarks, although intended to reassure, led to my internal retort, "No, they don't die on the table. They die when you take them off."

Dr. Blair called by phone and then introduced us in person to his ENT surgical colleague, Dr. Wilson. Like the team at Columbia-Presbyterian, the two of them would jointly perform the surgery. With both doctors Suzie and I discussed Dr. Barnet's partial-resection recommendation, which the Sinai physicians dismissed very quickly. Wilson, a warm, friendly man, expressed his personal and professional respect for Dr. Barnet, noting, as had other doctors, that they had enjoyed some time together on the tennis court. Following this expression of respect (which mostly seemed to indicate that a good time was had by all), Suzie challenged Dr. Wilson by referring to his quick dismissal of Barnet's recommendation. Wilson smiled and shrugged in response.

Dr. Blair stated in conclusion that he thought he could remove about 95% of the tumor. Of course he noted all the risks. I asked him, as I had Dr. Martin, whom he might consult with outside the city were he in my situation. He asked us what names we had. We mentioned Dr. Espinal in Pittsburgh and Blair simply said, "He's no longer there," leaving us to wonder if he had disappeared. At Dr. Gallagher's name, Blair nodded, with some evident reservation. When we mentioned Dr. Neria's name, Blair noted that they had worked together in the past (in Pittsburgh) and stated with clear admiration, "He's a good man." He also left us with the impression that, were we to consult with Dr. Neria, Blair himself suspected that we would be more likely to choose Neria for the surgery.

At the interview's end, Suzie, sensing a negative drift in Dr. Blair's remarks about the viability and effectiveness of surgery, again asked him if our children might be fatherless. He responded, "You have my hopes and my prayers." This answer, Suzie later mentioned several times, was simply not good enough.

That same afternoon I received a call from a resident working with Dr. Barnet. He informed me that in two days a large group of doctors at Sloan-Kettering would be having a conference on my case. He said they needed the original sets of films to digitize in order to hand out copies to the conference participants. He stated that they required the original films no later than noon the following day. I assumed that this development was the outcome of my conversation with Lydia from the administrator's office.

He Can Do Things No One Else Can

My first appointment the next day, day 34 of the magical mystery tour, was with Dr. Rief, the radiation oncologist for head and neck cancer at Beth Israel. He was reputed to be the best radiation oncologist for head and neck tumors in New York (i.e., in the world), the most knowledgeable, experienced, and clinically adept. He had worked for many years at Sloan-Kettering before moving to Beth Israel.

My appointment was for 9 A.M. but when we arrived we found that the receptionist with whom I had spoken the previous week had failed to enter the appointment in the computer. This omission would delay our being seen, as financial and insurance information needed to be entered and cleared. As it turned out, it was 11:35 by the time we were actually seen, and the films we were carrying had to be up at Memorial by noon (for digitizing). Additionally, I was scheduled to have an octreoscan (the nuclear medicine test) performed at noon, with a follow up scheduled for 4 P.M. as well as 11 A.M. the next day.

Thus I was agitated when we began our meeting with Dr. Rief. I immediately described the time situation to him and said I had expected to have a full consultation with him in the presence of my wife, who would have to leave momentarily to bring the films uptown. He said we could talk a bit right now but also offered to see me two days later to complete our discussion. In this, our first meeting, Dr. Rief stated that it was impossible to know how my tumor, given its extreme rarity, might respond to radiation. Despite his wealth of experience, he had not seen one like it. He indicated that, generally speaking, slow-growing tumors respond less well than fast-growing ones, because the latter were more likely to be "hit" in their growth cycles. He emphasized that there was much uncertainty. He asked my age (44), told me that there were only a few years' difference between us, and then said, "One hundred years from now we'll both be in the same place. But we don't know who will get there first." While this was no consolation under the circumstances, and it sounded like a line delivered many times before, I still appreciated his openly referring to my death. I mentioned that we were considering consulting with Dr. Neria in Boston, and Rief immediately said, "Good. *He can do things that no one else can.* . . . He wrote the chapter on skull-base surgery in our book" (one that he and Dr. Logan, also from Beth Israel, had coedited on head and neck cancer).

The long wait, the rush in the discussion, Suzie's leaving after only a few minutes, and Rief's reservations about the potential effectiveness of radiation in my case, all combined to leave me quite shaken, which was evident to Rief. He asked me how I was getting uptown—a question that momentarily surprised me—and when I indicated that I was going by cab, he said he would accompany me out of the building. We left his office, rode the elevator down, and walked through the lobby and revolving door. Facing the tumult of Union Square traffic, Dr. Rief gave me his beeper number and his home number and encouraged me to call if I had any questions. These gestures were very meaningful to me. Amid the endless waiting, the ordinary and extraordinary indifference and coldness of the world, the offer of contact was an anomaly.

Rief was not shielding himself from me but was instead opening himself to me in a direct and personal manner. He overtly identified with my situation and acknowledged the toll of the waiting and the doubt, the tension, and the proximity to death.

Perseverance and Serendipity

*I*dentification with my circumstances was more than
many could bear. Half an hour after seeing Dr. Rief,
while I sat in the waiting room at Sloan-Kettering prior to
my octreoscan, an older man began talking with me about
his condition (prostate cancer recurrence), my situation,
and the anticipated tests. As in other similar circumstances,
I was inclined to chat to pass the time. However, as also occurred on several other occasions, after brief summaries of
our respective conditions, the other patient abruptly ended
the conversation with, "I'm sure glad *I'm* not in *your* shoes."

Like all the other scans, the octreoscan required me to
be very still for an extended period. At times during these
tests, when my head was encased and clamped down in a

small, tight tunnel, I would think of certain things that would lead me to cry. This was an awkward but in some way pleasing experience, given my absolute restraint and corpse-like, physical rigidity. It was a small sign of life. In this particular instance, I lay still and tearful during the extended procedure only to learn (after an hour?) that the computers hadn't functioned properly and the whole thing had to be done over again.

That evening Suzie informed me that Dr. Neria had called from Boston. A formal and courteous man, he told her that, after viewing the films, he thought he could help us. An appointment was scheduled for five days later (Monday, October 18th, day 39). Neria suggested that we take a look at his Web site, which was impressive in several respects. It presented the consortium of doctors in Boston that Neria had organized for treatment of illness in the skull-base region. It listed all the doctors, their specialties, credentials, and experience. It contained descriptions and photographs of some of Neria's work with adults, and children with birth defects, along with some studies and data. It struck me as an attempt to be open, forthright, and informative, even though I could only glance at the materials. I waited anxiously to meet Dr. Neria in person.

The next evening a message was left on our home answering machine by Dr. Hughes, the radiation oncologist at Memorial Sloan-Kettering. She informed me of the recommendations that emerged from the large conference held that afternoon regarding my case. Radiation and chemotherapy were recommended; the partial resection via endoscopy was not. Hughes concluded by saying that I could also expect to hear from Dr. Barnet and Dr. Samuel. I was initially annoyed that this message was left on an answering machine. I was bothered by the fact that it was heard by Jacob, my nine-year-old son. However, recognizing the vagaries of making contact, I shrugged in resignation.

It was now the case that the recommendations of the Memorial and the Beth Israel teams coincided. Had they done so earlier, I might have proceeded without surgery. The doctors from these hospitals appeared to have the broadest and deepest experience, and I had been leaning in their direction. But my misgivings about Dr. Barnet were critical in my postponing a decision. Along with the delay in the pathology findings, these misgivings fortuitously permitted and encouraged further consultations. Were it not for the poor communication among Dr. Barnet, his colleagues, and me, I might not have kept searching as long as I did.

On a First-Name Basis

At the end of the week, Suzie and I went downtown to Beth Israel's ambulatory care center (on 14th Street and Union Square) to meet again with Dr. Rief, who said he preferred to be called Dan. He was the only doctor, of all we encountered, who wanted to be addressed by his first name. This suggested a desire on Rief's part to be less formal and distant, to be more personal. It conveyed an inclination to shift some of the standard features of doctor–patient relations. It was a gesture with which I was briefly uncomfortable. In fact I called Dan "Dr. Rief" a few times, and he laughed and teased me about this. I had an inclination to rely on the social expression of clearly demarcated roles and the acceptance and respect for authority they implied. Dan's strongly expressed preference, on the other hand, appeared to alter personal and professional boundaries and to disrupt the conventional hierarchy. As such, it was a risk he deemed worth taking, similar to his giving me his home phone number. Conceivably permitting more intimate, relaxed, and personal contact, it was an attempt to level the playing field. It encouraged greater familiarity and a sense of collaboration.

As our consultation progressed, I told Dan that I had had the octreoscan but had not yet received the results. While we sat there, he called the nuclear medicine department at Memorial, asked to speak to Dr. Saha (whom Dan knew from his 10 years at that hospital), and reported the results to me: negative, the tumor did not take up the radio-isotope. I was prepared for this outcome—friends had done a literature search that provided scant evidence for the effectiveness of octreotides even should I test positive. The whole idea had seemed to be a measure of the weakness of the chemotherapy options. Dan's phone call, though, was another example of his readiness to act on my behalf and his openness and desire to keep me well informed. It wasn't until six days later that I was told of the results by someone from the Memorial staff.

Dan, Suzie, and I discussed the questions pertaining to the radiation, given the size, location, and pathology of the tumor. Dan was admittedly skeptical of accomplishing much and indicated that he thought we had less than a 50–50 chance of eliminating the cancer. He said he "wouldn't be selling any tickets to this as a demonstration of the effectiveness of radiation."

When I mentioned our upcoming consultation with Dr. Neria, Dan reiterated his respect for him. He took his own book on head and neck cancer (a heavy volume) off the shelf and opened it to Dr. Neria's chapter on skull-base surgery. He thought that if anyone might have seen one or two tumors similar to mine, it would be Dr. Neria. Dan also offered, if I wished, for him and Dr. Logan (the head and neck oncology surgeon at Beth Israel) to speak with Neria following our consultation in Boston. He said that he and Dr. Logan might disagree with Dr. Neria and might still recommend against surgery, but they would go over all the risks and anatomical details with him. I was again impressed with Dan's openness and willingness to act on my behalf, to confer, in my presence if I desired, even if doing so involved my seeking surgery at another institution. His behavior was a notable exception to the pattern of professional distance and institutional confinement I otherwise encountered. He was prepared to become personally involved.

Later that day I called both Dr. Barnet and Dr. Samuel in an unsuccessful effort to speak with them. I was still trying to follow up on the conference at Memorial. I left a message with Dr. Samuel's receptionist that I would like to meet with Dr. Samuel in person. I wanted to hear his specific final recommendations. That evening I had a pelvic and abdomen CT scan (which had been ordered by Samuel) to check for possible metastases.

Help! I Need Somebody

Over the weekend we went up to Westchester, where my son Jacob had a soccer game, and good friends of ours joined us at the field. At the time, it was still quite plausible to me that I might die soon. I went for a brief walk with my friend Kenny, a child psychologist and psychoanalyst. The field was adjacent to a marina beside which I later sat, watching boats slowly entering and leaving. Kenny and I wandered away from the field and toward the water. I worried aloud about my death and the difficulties my wife and children would face and said I wanted those people who I thought could help, like Kenny, to know that their help and presence were important to me.

With difficulty, as I got choked up, I told Kenny that I loved him and his family. I also said I thought he had a special facility, an ability to establish a rapport with kids, something I had observed many times, particularly when he spoke with Jacob. He played with him, put him at ease, chatted. I knew it would be difficult, with significant limitations, but I asked him to help look after my kids if I couldn't, to the extent it was possible. At first he seemed a little bewildered, asking if I expected to have the surgery right away in Boston. I said no, I was sure there would be some delay, some waiting period. Kenny then sought to reassure me; he said it was very easy to talk with my kids. He also said, alluding to his longstanding appreciation of my older son's, Jacob's, intelligence, that he fully expected to be present at our celebration (a decade hence) of Jacob's graduation from Harvard. While said in a generous and warm spirit, this remark was dislocating and saddening. Unintentionally, it prompted me to imagine an event at which I would not be present and deepened my fear of Jacob's being fatherless.

Not Just Anybody

*F*orty days into the search for a treatment with a good and convincing chance of success, Suzie and I took an early flight up to Boston. We were driven to the airport by a friend, Ellen, who had herself recently engaged in a struggle with breast cancer.

When we arrived at Brigham and Women's Hospital and Children's Hospital—they are interconnected in a large web of medical institutions—we had some time and ate a small lunch in the restaurant in the lobby. Many hospitals are now visually indistinguishable in some respects, having areas that are mall-like (with chain drug and food shops), with architecture designed to be impressive, to give a large sense of scale, but strikingly empty and artificial in feeling.

(This is my impression of new additions at Columbia-Presbyterian, Mount Sinai, Beth Israel, and Brigham.) There is a reach for monumentality and grandeur with an absence of decorative detail or uniqueness, resulting in shallowness and sterility. Some of the older remnant sections, like that through which we went to Dr. Neria's office, have a distinctive quaintness which feels much more human.

After eating in the lobby, we went to the children's science store that lay behind an elaborate and whimsical marble run. Inside I came across detailed anatomical renderings of the head and brain. With five minutes before our appointment and with Suzie coaxing me away, I studied the images with attempted diligence and intensity, aware of the absurdity but still hoping to orient myself better. At different moments during the preceding weeks, I had even considered purchasing light boards in order to be able to view the films and train myself in the anatomy. My thirst for knowledge was understandable, as was my desire to cope with what was almost an everyday experience of looking at pictures I could not read. Of course I realized that I couldn't provide myself with the training and experience that would make such an endeavor meaningful. I could not develop an independence of judgment with regard to the appearance of the scans. All I could do was scrutinize the various qualities of a doctor's interpretation.

Dr. Neria's office was run by his wife, who was gracious, warm, and plainspoken. When we arrived she gave me an extensive questionnaire to fill out, which included questions associated with my psychological well-being (What was I most looking forward to? How satisfied was I with my work?) and with my personal attachments (What were the names of my children?). No other office had solicited such information, which, simply by being asked, left the impression that I was being attended to in an unusually intense and personal manner.

Dr. Neria, a trim, relatively small, balding man around 60, wore a bow tie and had something of an Old World manner. (I had learned of his European birthplace through his Web site.) Calm and courteous, he began with a meticulous physical exam. The implements that he used he drew from a handheld case that he brought into the room. He was the only doctor I saw for whom this was true. I had the feeling that he cared for his tools meticulously. On the ceiling of the consulting room he had placed a poster of the Rockies, in recognition of his patients' posture during the physicals—and perhaps also as an allusion to the terrain examined.

Dr. Neria started our discussion by noting that he was aware from our phone exchanges that there was a divergence of opinion about how to proceed in my case. I mentioned several quite contradictory perspectives. He laughed and said "19 doctors, 19 opinions." He said that what was most important, though, was that a doctor's recommendations make sense to me. He looked at the films with us and as he did so I was immediately impressed with his grasp of what he saw. He was capable of visualizing the tumor in three dimensions, he identified things clearly, and he conveyed to us what he perceived. Where there was uncertainty about how to read something, he described the various alternatives and gave his judgment with reasons. He noted, for example, that one area near an eye, where it appeared that the tumor had broken through some bone, was more likely a congenital defect, given its shape, size, and direction. The bone curled, and there was no evidence of a "mushrooming" of the tumor. He said he thought the tumor did not involve the brain, that it had not fully broken through the clivus. He showed that two somewhat separate parts to the tumor were visible: two small balloons, with some tissue and bone incorporated between them. He was the only doctor to point out any of these things and to describe them.

Dr. Neria said he thought he could remove 100% of the visible tumor (again, he was the only physician who said this), but he would be unable to get the necessary 10% margin around the tumor. He thought the surgery would take 7 to 10 hours but might extend to 11 or 12. He indicated that radiation following surgery would still be a necessity. He noted that patients often found the radiation and the recovery from it more onerous than the surgery. Dr. Neria added that, during the surgery, some bone would have to be reconstructed with titanium mesh. (Besides being a skull-base surgeon, Dr. Neria was also trained as a plastic surgeon.) He stated that he thought chemotherapy at this point would be purely speculative.

In response to my questions, Dr. Neria said that he would not have recommended surgery were the pathology different (e.g., an adenocarcinoma) and that he had seen two tumors with similar pathology (he was also alone in this), one of which had been larger and had penetrated the brain, but both of which he had been able to remove. It was his impression that the tumor was of a kind that could be extracted in its entirety. If he encountered problems that posed too great a risk, he would proceed no further. In regard to the pathology, he noted that the implications of several of the stains were unknown. He said that formerly this tumor would have been indistinguishable from the more common esthesioneuroblastoma. However, despite there being little experience with the distinctions, he thought my type of tumor had a slightly better prognosis. He said that with surgery and radiation there was an 80% to 85% chance of no recurrence. Dr. Neria added that prior to surgery he would have an angiogram performed in order to assess the blood supply to the tumor and to better plan the surgery. No one else had mentioned the use of this procedure.

Neria said he would perform the entire surgery himself, with a frontal approach through the face, meaning that no brain contents would be touched. A neurosurgeon, an innovative and renowned doctor, would stand by, but Dr. Neria did not believe he would be needed.

Toward the end of our interview, Neria indicated that were we to go ahead with the surgery with him, we would have to wait several weeks before he would be able to do it. I asked if I might experience in the interim some of the symptoms many of the doctors had asked me about: blurring or loss of vision; diminished sensation in my face; headaches or loss of hearing. Neria laughed and said, "Oh, you will," signaling that most patients eventually experience the symptoms they are warned of. I enjoyed his levity, as well as the fact that I had no such symptoms. I asked if he would speak with Dr. Logan and Dr. Rief in New York, and he answered, "Yes, certainly," although, perhaps anticipating that they might differ with him, he added, "But the decision is yours."

Each of Neria's answers to our many questions confirmed my strong initial impression. After only 20 minutes (I had glanced down at my watch) I felt convinced of Dr. Neria's expertise and skill. His behavior was not notable for its warmth or personal visibility, but neither was he brusque or impatient. He had been respectful and thorough, as well as playful at times, and he seemed to appreciate the benefit of an actively engaged patient.

On the flight back to New York, Suzie and I tried to calm and measure our perceptions and emotions. We were feeling optimistic, yet we also knew that such feelings could be short-lived.

One thing that struck me with considerable force was that I had come upon Dr. Neria through personal and nonmedical channels (my patient Roland and my acquaintance Denise). It was evident that he specialized in the surgery I needed and had more experience than anyone else I had spoken with. Yet no one with whom I consulted had volunteered his name. Despite their conscious efforts at openness, even the members of the Beth Israel team had not suggested a consultation in Boston, although Dr. Neria and his expertise were well known to both Drs. Logan and Rief. That the Beth Israel team did not initiate a referral was, I believe, an error of omission, an unintentional consequence of their limited range of vision.

The following day I called Dr. Neria's office. I had decided to go ahead with the surgery to be performed by him and asked that it be scheduled as soon as possible. I did this before I received a phone call that afternoon from Dan (Dr. Rief). He said that both he and Dr. Logan had spoken with Dr. Neria, and they wholeheartedly recommended that I proceed with the surgery. He wanted to make sure what they had to say was clear and emphatic: they were unequivocally recommending that I go ahead. They had discussed the anatomical details and it appeared to them that with Dr. Neria it was worth the risk. Dr. Neria had convinced them that he could accomplish something significant. Dan said,

"Even if he can't do what he believes he can, it will probably still be of benefit." When I received this call I was in my
office with Suzie and was momentarily elated. Although I
had reached a similar conclusion, it was significant that Dr.
Logan and Dan had reversed their opinions about the advisability of surgery. Their efforts on my behalf were of
tremendous value in the subsequent weeks as I waited for
the date of surgery and endured doubts and misgivings.

He Will Operate on
Anyone Who Lets Him

A principal source of my misgivings was a phone call I received the following morning from Dr. Barnet. I had been told I would hear from him following Memorial's conference on my case and the change in recommendations. I had left a message the previous week and he had tried contacting me. He called at 8 A.M. on my cell phone, just as I was trying to get the kids out the door and on their way to school. I attempted to find a quiet alcove for the conversation. I stood just inside the front door to our apartment.

"We've been playing telephone tag," he began.

"Yes."

133

"What's up? What's on your mind?"

"I wanted to know about the change in treatment recommendations. What were the considerations involved?"

From here on Barnet sounded annoyed and impatient,
and he began attributing to me motives that I believe had
much more to do with him than with me.

"David, you want a definitive answer! A definitive answer
in a situation where there is none!"

"Dr. Barnet, I am not interested in a definitive answer
where there is none. I recognize there are limits to what can be
known. I am interested in understanding the process though,
the considerations, what would lead to a change of mind."

"There is nothing definitive here! . . . The recommendation, the consensus, is radiation and chemotherapy. That's
it! . . . It's what I would tell a family member. Radiation and
chemotherapy."

"Dr. Samuel has told me that there is no clear chemotherapy in my case."

"That's for you to discuss with Dr. Samuel."

"I understand that, but he has said he doesn't know what
to prescribe. It has bearing on the recommendation. It's not
your domain, I know that. I also haven't heard from him."

"Well, you *are* my patient . . . and it's important that the
whole team communicates with you. . . . If you don't mind
my asking, who else have you consulted with?"

"I have consulted with Dr. Logan and Dr. Rief at Beth
Israel, who initially recommended chemotherapy and radiation. I've consulted with Dr. Martin at Columbia, Dr. Blair
at Sinai, and Dr. Neria in Boston. I was not particularly convinced by Dr. Martin or Dr. Blair, who recommended surgery, but when I . . ."

Dr. Barnet interrupted me.

"*They would all operate on anyone who let them!*"

"You feel that way about Dr. Neria as well?"

"Yes. He will operate on anyone who lets him. . . . This is *not* a surgical cancer! Let me tell you something, David. When it comes to surgeons, their egos get involved. And they will go ahead and do surgery when they shouldn't. . . . I don't know how many surgeries in this area any of these doctors has performed, but I did three in the past two weeks. I do more than anybody else, and this is *not* a surgical cancer!"

"It's your sense that it's just too dangerous?"

"It's the whole gestalt of the thing, if I may use that word with you. It's the whole gestalt. . . . This is not a surgical cancer! That's what I would tell a member of my family. . . . Let us know what you decide."

"I will."

The conversation was rapid and intense. Dr. Barnet sounded fiercely angry, even belligerent. He may be an excellent surgeon, but his conduct toward me left much to be desired. His impugning the character of the other surgeons was very unsettling and struck me as quite unwarranted. He was apparently irritated that his authority was not simply accepted; he evidently preferred a docile patient. It appeared that to Dr. Barnet we had become adversaries. I remembered Barnet's avowed openness to uncertainty and attachment to empiricism, which now seemed to be transformed into shut-the-door assertions. Of course, a person's articulated position can be quite inconsistent with his or her actual practice; the proclaimed attitude may be a reaction against a characteristic tendency. But when it came to talking about surgeons' egos or the need for definitive answers, the pot did seem to be calling the kettle black.

Yet this conversation continued to bother me. The surgery I had scheduled with Neria was several weeks away, and during that time many of Barnet's phrases and pronouncements reverberated in my head. I could readily marshal the instances of what I took to be his poor thinking, his impulsiveness, and his psychological naivete. And yet Dr. Barnet had come so strongly recommended; he had been represented as *the* expert in this area, the person who did the most surgery, the surgeon who was the most technically proficient. He was at a renowned institution with supposedly incomparable experience and authority, and that institution had held a conference on my case out of which had emerged a recommendation that did not include surgery.

While Dr. Neria had impressed me, there were ways I could construe what I knew of his history and experience, as well as what I knew of people in general, to grow fearful that he might be too willing to perform a surgery that was exceedingly risky. He had been doing surgery for many years and had engaged at an earlier time in salvage operations—in operations to buy time, which led to progress in technique, but which were not curative. If I let my skepticism go to its extreme, I might focus on hypothetical motives having to do with his own prejudices and desires, things which might obscure his vision. Yet I never found these doubts convincing. I believed he was reliable and a person of integrity. I leaned on Logan's and Rief's recommendation, and I trusted my experience and perceptions in Neria's presence.

What You Don't Want

After several phone calls I was able to arrange to meet again with Dr. Samuel. At our meeting he explained the delay by indicating he had not assumed that I wanted to speak with him again in person, and he asked me to be more explicit with his receptionist in the future. Although I had been explicit in my requests and told him so, I nevertheless thought his handling of the evident misunderstanding was courteous and professional. When we met it was in a different building than we had had our original meeting, although I had not been informed of this change by his receptionist and it entailed quite a bit of scurrying at the last moment. This new space was a richly decorated suite of offices, where the waiting area appeared modeled on a

Japanese tea garden, with lots of running water and partitions. The goal was undoubtedly a soothing and calming environment, although, in my limited observation, it was a Disney World–like stage set, a kitsch surface patina meant to counter intense anxiety.

Over two hours late, Dr. Samuel began our consultation by saying, "I hear you've been traveling." To which Suzie and I responded in amusing unison, "Who told you that?" Dr. Samuel chose to avoid a direct answer: "Well, you have a lot of friends. A lot of people have called about you." Samuel then gave a description of my situation but seemed to be speaking from a perspective that had been colored by a communication from Dr. Barnet; that is, he was emphasizing and belaboring the fact that there was no definitive answer.

I broke in: "Dr. Samuel, you mentioned earlier about my traveling. I want to let you know about that. We've consulted with Dr. Neria in Boston and are planning to go ahead with the surgery with him. I spoke with Dr. Barnet a few days ago. This may be neither here nor there to you, but several times Dr. Barnet has acted in a peremptory manner with me. (In my obsessiveness I later looked up *peremptory* in the dictionary to make sure I had used it correctly.) I have asked simple questions and Dr. Barnet has responded dismissively. At one point he chose to say, "You and I are two different kinds of people," with my falling in some purported group that continues to ask questions rather than simply finding and accepting the best authority. . . . I just wanted a professional opinion from Dr. Barnet, as I do from you. He repeatedly suggested I wanted a definitive answer when none existed. That isn't so. What I would like is an understanding of what went into the final treatment recommendations."

Dr. Samuel appeared uncomfortable and anxious in response to my statement (although he did before, as well). I had tried to be measured, but it was difficult to contain my distress and anger. Although I had anticipated that Samuel wouldn't comment on Dr. Barnet, I wanted to let him know Barnet had upset me. Dr. Samuel reacted to my remarks by more openly attempting to describe the process of their decision making.

"It's true we've waffled on your case several times. I've changed my mind more than once. I've thought there was no basis on which to prescribe any medication and so none should be given. But I've also thought: You're young, your body can probably handle it, why not try something? We looked carefully at the films and discussed the options. Larry, the pathologist, was present and he offered the thought, entirely subjective, but this was his 'feel,' that there may be intermediate elements in the tumor, some growing more rapidly. This was entirely subjective—it would never be written in a report. I spoke with one neurosurgeon who thought surgery should be attempted. We went back and forth in every area. There's no clear path on how to proceed. I would, I suppose, prescribe something. It's very difficult, very hard, you know. . . . You and I are about the same age . . . the children . . . and all . . ."

Here Dr. Samuel trailed off. The reference to our age and children, an overt non sequitur, was revealing. Several other doctors also appeared to struggle with their tendency to identify with me and the powerful urge to do something.

I asked several more questions of Dr. Samuel that followed from my decision to go ahead with Dr. Neria. I asked him what he knew of Dr. Neria. He replied, "I know he's one of the best, one of the five best perhaps, for surgery in the skull base. But I've never been in the OR with him. What you don't want is someone going in there and hacking around." I found this remark less than illuminating. Internally I reacted with the highly articulate, "Duh!" whereas externally I mumbled, "It's not my impression that's what Dr. Neria would be doing."

Samuel also noted that an important aspect of a doctor's job is picking his patients, knowing whom to treat and when. His reference to being selective in this manner reinforced for me the importance of Dr. Neria's confidence and clarity. Samuel remarked that what applied to the chemotherapy was true for the surgery, as well: "It would be different if you were 60 or more, but you're young and will probably come through the surgery okay."

At another point, when discussing postoperative treatment, I indicated that I would probably be seeing Dr. Rief for the radiation but wondered if it would be possible for Dr. Samuel to do the chemotherapy, as everyone said he was the best. He answered, "Logistically it would be too difficult because the chemotherapy would probably require several inpatient stays. But to tell you the truth, and not to diminish what I do, once I decide on the medication, I write the prescriptions and the nurses give the injections. It's the radiation that will require some hands-on technical skill, and I love working with Dan." Samuel said he would be available at any point for further consultation.

Awkward and tense, indirect as well as straightforward, the conversation was yet another fragment in the continuously turbulent struggle for access and understanding.

What I Deserve

After we left this meeting I had a thought which I had consistently repressed, kept down and away, nipped in the bud on all earlier occasions: "I deserve to have this work out. I deserve to live." I had previously efficiently rejected this thought as irrelevant and, in reality, a form of superstition. When others commented to me in this vein, I would shake my head and say, "I don't think it works that way." After all, I did not think I deserved this to happen at all. It had *nothing* to do with being deserving or not. It was my view that Nature does not act in moral terms. Neither does it take prisoners. What we call Nature—ranging from the activity of things at a microbiological level to volcanoes or earthquakes or events in the universe—occurs in utter

141

disregard of individual human life. Even putting it in such terms ("disregard") appears to suggest a more purposeful interaction than actually exists. Illness can strike in an entirely arbitrary manner as far as our selves are concerned.

While I recognize that we are meaning-creating animals, our impulse to invent meanings can be harmful—demonizing, idealizing, obfuscating, or simplifying. Just the thought that, because this has happened to me I will necessarily try to make meanings of it, seems like an entrapment. The making of meanings is, of course, quite different from something being inherent. It may provide some scope for choice, may be adaptive, and may have clear survival value—but so do skepticism and realism.

Yet the predictable question just doesn't go away: What *does* this have to do with me? We get used to believing that what happens to us personally has something to do with our selves. We want to foster the feeling, to believe this, to make it so. Such thoughts and feelings are a means of countering our experience of powerlessness, of the accidental, of the chaotic. But it is all too easy to fail to differentiate between those things that have something to do with our selves and those that don't.

So, my answer to the question at the time, unsatisfying as it may be, was . . . Nothing. The illness has *nothing* to do with me as I existed before it occurred. It was not something meant specifically for me, like a message or warning or punishment; nor was it prescribed for my moral betterment. In retrospect, I prefer not to subdue my experience by such means, to hold it aloft and remove it from contact with the earth, as Hercules did to defeat earthbound Antaeus. Rather, I imagine that it will wriggle away, change color and shape, continue to intrude and influence, whatever the means I use to grapple with its presence.

For a time, even an extended time, a malignant growth in the center of one's skull is entirely usurping—it overwhelms and obliterates, permits virtually nothing else to exist. There are impulses both to accept and to escape its dominance and centrality, simultaneously to embrace and to evade its crushing intensity. It is not satisfying to temporize or qualify its prominence. It felt like the air I breathed, the atmosphere in which I lived, and the city that surrounded me, despite the fact that it resided within my head.

The thought, "I deserve to survive," led to a brief moment of enjoyable illogic, like rooting for the home team.

Beckett wrote, "It's impossible I should have a mind and I have one." A mind that, given its remarkable perceptual and cognitive capacities, often persists in functioning out of accord with reality and beyond experience, forming and clinging to wantonly erroneous conceptions.

Now These Days Are Gone,
I'm Not So Self-Assured

The meeting with Dr. Samuel occurred on Friday, October 22nd, and brought to a conclusion the round of major consultations that I had prior to the surgery, which was scheduled for November 15th. In the intervening weeks I met, at the suggestion of one of my medical friends, with a neurooncologist at Columbia-Presbyterian. Our conversation was directed mostly to postoperative care and concerns. I also met with an ophthalmologist, who confirmed that my eyesight had not been affected, and with the medical oncologist on the Beth Israel team.

I had several weeks of waiting and apprehension. During that period I wasn't seeing my patients, although I did contact them and convey my plans: I told them that I thought I would be returning to work in January (possibly only for a brief time) and then taking another two-month medical leave owing to anticipated radiation treatment. I said I would contact them in the second week of December to let them know about my plans more definitively. Most patients wanted to know some details of my treatment, although only one asked about the specific date of the surgery and the name of the hospital where it was taking place. While I did answer the question, the request brought forth a desire to protect my privacy along with recognition that the patient's curiosity and impulse to care were natural.

I had arranged for colleagues to be available, on the phone and in person, either for my patients to see in my absence or for any inquiries they might have about my medical situation and status. Several did call to inquire, and a few sought appointments with the covering therapists. At various times during the autumn months, facets of my relations with patients would come into focus or be illuminated— most commonly, their dependence on me and my dependence on them (emotionally, professionally, financially). I also felt at times that I was, of course, dispensable and replaceable. But for the most part these attachments receded, and I was occupied and preoccupied elsewhere.

In the weeks before the surgery Suzie worked out a schedule for who would be with our children while we were in Boston. Her mom was going to come in from Rochester and be the continuous presence in our home, but with plenty of support from family and friends, and in particular from Mary, who had helped care for all our children since they were infants. The arrangements Suzie made were formidable and resourceful, which didn't stop me from pestering her until they were finalized. I knew our children would be as well taken care of as was possible under the circumstances. My parents and sister would be coming up to Boston for the day of the surgery and the following day. When they returned, they would help with the children. Suzie's brother, who lived in San Francisco, also came to Boston. He had asked me if I wanted him to come and I had replied, "I'd feel safer if you were there." If something went wrong, if there were complications, I felt reassured that Joe, a doctor in the family, would be present.

Of course I did worry about the possible complications: blindness and stroke, and some things leading to death, or a semblance thereof. I remained concerned that some of the best doctors around had recommended against the surgery, that Sloan-Kettering, as an institution, did as well. I would offer myself the challenge: How is it that I think I can judge the situation better than they? I had answers: my impression of Dr. Neria; Logan's and Rief's support; my perception of Barnet. But this did not eliminate the questions or the anxiety.

In those weeks I went to my studio most days but didn't work on anything new. I revised older work and mounted recent paintings on panels. Although it felt incongruous, I arranged for a gallery director to visit my studio. Since June I had been working on paintings in which I destroyed and transformed books. I ripped out their pages, carved deeply into them; I pasted fragments from one text into and on top of another. I doused the remnants with oil, shellac, polyurethane, and wood stain. I stuck pieces of bark inside their gouged interiors and around their borders. I poured, brushed, dripped, and splashed the paint. The books appeared as though they had been decomposed and reconstructed, dismantled and welded, eviscerated and cast in lead. I sometimes removed the books from the paper and wood panels placed beneath them and then remounted them elsewhere in the painting, leaving behind their imprints in the original paper, their ghost images. Some of the paintings looked as though a fire had been raging over the materials. Some looked like archaeological sites with fossilized remains. The paintings had passages that resembled shards preserved through accidental processes, surviving bone and book fragments still imperiled by uncontrollable natural and historical forces.

In sympathy with more than one modernist tradition, I had been in a mood for some time, well before my diagnosis, in which I was not interested in making an image or a representation, a picture, something that hung on a wall, sedately or not (or so I said to myself every now and then). Rather, I worked on paintings that were less images than the thing itself, the residue of actions. Carving in and out of books, and then painting over and into them, gave me the feeling of life emerging from something preexistent, life embedded in past moments but charging through them like an electric current into the present. It was as though I carved flesh and blood from the books or drew them out of the texts and into organic fragments, like the pieces of bark. The presences that emerged from these procedures felt as though they existed on the edge of discontinuity, dissolution, and death. There was exhilaration in finding precarious form, urgent movements teetering on disintegration.

I had sought ways of working which embodied my constantly renewed and unsatisfied craving for structure and intelligibility, as well as my destructiveness, my rejection of order and organization. The means I used grew out of an

erratically conscious, ever-unfolding, experimental process. Sometimes it occurred to me that the eviscerated and
painted books could be emblems of consciousness, or individuality, or collective and personal treasures. But whatever
they were, they appeared as ruins. The manner of the
books' use explicitly captured my hostility to definitions
and representations held as sacred, my episodic but intense
disappointment and disillusionment with words, my despair at the pretenses associated with culture, and my admiration and love for some of its fragments. I identified with
the different processes that both effaced and secured, de-
faced and preserved. The vigorous, iconoclastic attacks on
texts, the manipulation and coercion of their contents, felt
like desperate and vain efforts to get inside, to be inside, to
be a part of, to grasp. The violation and profaning of the
books were coupled with a handling designed to open the
manuscripts and unfold their capacity for structure and
beauty.

These works also came into being as a response to my
impression of the contemporary context for painting,
which is really no singular context of significance, but a
multitude of insubstantial, fragile, or fictitious part-con-
texts. My sense is that contemporary painting or visual art is
cut off, is virtually without significant function or influence. In its various radical or conservative postures, all it
does is preach to the converted (or offer to enhance their
investments). Political, economic, and social realities operate independently from the artistic sphere; the diversity and
incoherence of these pieces of reality readily shatter any
consistent or stable aesthetic. There is thus a wide variety
of technical virtuosities for a host of aesthetics; there is a
plethora of styles or postures, but each having the status

equivalent of a perfume. There is no center and no periphery. The cultural context is fragmented and faceted in ways that make analytical cubism look relatively sedate, stable, and organized. We are in the midst of a continuous disorganization and disintegration, a tidal wave of styles and traditions flooding a defunct structure, one that has already collapsed into either chaos or temporary islands on the brink of being submerged. The collapse has its virtues, although they tend not to be conducive to an attentive and deep aesthetic gaze.

Unlike my work as a psychotherapist, my painting has given relatively free reign to my destructive feelings, which are very close neighbors to, sometimes even indistinguishable from, my creative ones. When painting, I can seek, and fully permit, the egregious and harmful. My concern for an object is much more willingly and freely overcome. I don't have to make concessions, to be diplomatic, temperate, realistic, or to engage in strategies for coaxing others. There is no need to inhibit my appetites, my voraciousness, my love of accident, my need to recover from order and organization. There is no conventional role to tolerate or to resist, no external authority, no obligatory routines.

In psychotherapy, by contrast, there is the relinquishing of an exclusively self-willed aesthetic. There is an immediate and spontaneous counter to solipsism, a relief from personal preoccupation, and a direct and considerable responsibility to another human being. I can't, by any means, shape and deform to my heart's delight. Another person, with his or her own aesthetic and will, is the focus, although both people emerge in whatever creativity takes place.

During the several weeks of waiting for my surgery, the process of drying a few earlier paintings and mounting them on panels was slow, quiet, manual; it involved little thought and was a solace.

These Little Town Blues

We went up to Boston on Thursday, November 11th, for the preoperative testing, which included a CT scan. Dr. Neria mentioned to me that this would be done without dye. Of course, in this instance, the technician wanted to administer the dye, until I objected and she checked the records. She also fitted me for a plastic helmet (with numerous apertures) that I would wear during the surgery. Once it was placed on my head I was asked to hold up both hands with two of my central fingers attached. The technician then giggled and said, "Star Trek!"

On Friday I was scheduled to have an angiogram, but it wasn't until that morning that the procedure was fully explained to me. A catheter was inserted in my thigh and dexterously manipulated through my upper torso into my skull and into my brain. As Dr. Azov performed the procedure, he described to me what was happening. Dye was injected into the catheter and traveled into the blood vessels of my head. He would say, for example, "You will have a warm feeling coursing through your right eye," and moments later I would feel the fluid moving there.

The goal was to identify clearly the blood supply to the tumor and see if it would present difficulties for the surgery. If the latter was the case, Dr. Azov would attempt to embolize (cut off) the blood supply of one or more vessels. As it turned out, the blood supply was quite limited and no embolization was required. Dr. Neria came down to view the films and confirmed this finding. Azov showed me the many pictures on the screens hanging from the room's ceiling, and I was amazed to watch the liquids flow through the network of vessels in my brain. I was dazzled by the picture show and the technology. I remained in the recovery room for six hours following the procedure. Suzie and I then flew home to spend the weekend with Jacob, Judah, and Isaiah.

Saying Good-Bye

*P*rior to my leaving, several people called or came by. My friend Jerry told me to kick ass and take names. He and Eric, on separate occasions, said they would drive up to visit later in the week. I trembled in response, saying, "I'll be looking forward to it," hoping there *would* be somebody to visit. Ina, neighbor and physician, stopped by, and when I told her the results of the angiogram she mused aloud, "Maybe this will turn out okay."

Saul called Sunday afternoon. At our last meeting the preceding week I had said, "I don't think I'm gonna die," countering the possibility with a carefully considered opinion, a wish, an assertion with a shudder close behind it. Saul had concluded the session by saying, "Give it your best shot." Of course I was doing that, although by the time this point had arrived I felt it was no longer a matter of my will. I was putting my life in someone else's hands. When Saul called the day before the surgery, I told him of the angiogram results and remarked that the test should probably have been part of the diagnostic process. It wasn't, I assumed, because it would have been too costly. Saul expressed delight in the results of the angiogram and conveyed encouragement.

Saul's call, which was a surprise, reminded me of another moment, one during Judah's illness. About 12 hours after Judah had been transferred to NYU, I called Saul. Toward the end of our brief conversation, feeling that my child was on the edge of death, I said, "Saul, if you can . . . and it means something . . . pray for him." Saul had answered, "That goes without saying." Against the background of disciplined reserve, his remark, like the phone call the day before my surgery and one on the day I was discharged from the hospital, expressed the depth of his personal caring and involvement.

Several people told me they would be thinking of me during my surgery, which was expected to last 7 to 10 hours. Some friends mentioned they would pray for me, at times adding something about their own skepticism regarding its effectiveness. Such remarks comforted me, knowing others were aware of the danger and cared. There were many warm gestures from people I knew (from those who were close and some who were fairly distant acquaintances) which moved me deeply. My experience belied the rhetoric that sometimes surrounds us and is often addressed to the anonymity and coldness of contemporary urban life.

On Sunday Suzie's mom arrived midday, and Jacob was scheduled to go off to a soccer game with our friend Kenny just a little while before we left. Saying good-bye to him in the hall by the elevator, we both began to cry, something Jacob and I had not done together in the preceding two months. I think it was very hard or, more accurately, impossible for Jacob to open himself to the intensity of emotion and the fear. Knowing this, he chose to assume things would be okay. Jacob also chose, for the most part, not to talk about what was going on, either with me or with others. As we parted, I silently affirmed to myself, "I will see him again . . . I will see him again."

The surgery was scheduled for 7 A.M. on Monday, November 15th. Suzie and I arrived at the hospital at 5:30.

Street Fight

I awoke in the ICU many hours later, with an oxygen mask, among other things, over my face. Suzie was there to tell me that the surgery was more successful than Dr. Neria had hoped. After spending seven hours inside my head, he was able to tell her that he had removed the entire tumor cleanly, with a 10% margin in all areas but two: at the clivus and in the sphenoid sinus.

He described the complicated multistage procedure. The incision on my face went across the full breadth of the bottom of my nose, up along its right side to the bridge, and then across the bridge, into the corner of both eyes, then up to the lower edge of both eyebrows and along the brow bottom for about a quarter of an inch. He had peeled back the soft tissue and broken through bones on the right side of my face. As one friend playfully remarked, "He parked your nose in your ear!" Making the incision in the tumor, removing its contents, and carefully peeling away its exterior was tenderly accomplished. Dr. Neria then carved a right angle into the clivus and removed what he could by scraping. The intraoperational report consists of eight pages, single-spaced.

Suzie said I looked like someone who had been in a street fight—and lost. But one way or another, my appearance notwithstanding, I had survived, and it was likely that I would continue to do so for a while.

These Vagabond Shoes

*M*y recovery from the surgery was uneventful and without complications. I spent one week in the hospital (with Suzie beside me on a cot) and then several weeks at home. I was exhilarated: My efforts had borne fruit and I had made the right decision. Dr. Logan at Beth Israel, whom I saw for most of my postoperative care, repeated many times his surprise and pleasure at Dr. Neria's work. Laced with what sounded like a bit of envy and professional competitiveness, he marveled at the surgery he had initially recommended against: "You could have come back paralyzed or blind or both. . . . This kind of thing couldn't have been done a couple of years ago. . . . In fact I didn't think it could be done now. . . . You're a courageous man. . . . I'm very glad you went for broke." Perhaps it was a small measure of my denial, but I had been convinced of my odds with Dr. Neria after 20 minutes with the man. If I had been gambling, it was with calculation and caution. A year after the surgery, my son Jacob gave voice to one pole on the spectrum of denial: "I was never really worried or scared. . . . It was just a matter of finding the right doctor."

Still looming, however, was the next stage—determining what kind of radiation to have and where. The process in this instance differed considerably from that which had preceded it. I consulted only two doctors. Although their opinions differed, there were two reasonably good options, each with a promising prognosis. Following the successful surgery, the tumor's pathology was clearer and effective treatment was thought likely.

From prior experience, I trusted and respected Dan. He was the radiation oncologist with whom, if I stayed in New York, I would proceed. However, Dan, Dr. Neria, and others had mentioned the possibility of proton-beam radiation, which was available only in Boston and California. It was reported to be less dangerous to surrounding tissue than conventional photon-beam radiation, as the proton beams could be controlled to terminate at a specific spot whereas photon-beam radiation diffused gradually over space. Because of this, higher doses of proton-beam radiation could be delivered, as it was less necessary to protect adjacent structures. The proton beam and its effectiveness were still under study, but it was thought to be particularly useful with certain types of tumors.

Despite my limited energy following the surgery, I wanted to be clear about this option too. So I consulted with Dr. O'Brien in Boston. In response to his request, I gave him a detailed summary of the information regarding my prior care. In turn, he sent me an article he had coauthored regarding proton-beam radiation and chemotherapy treatment for my tumor type. Suzie and I made one more trip to Boston, which we coordinated with a follow-up visit to Dr. Neria. Time was of the essence, as it was generally agreed that I should start radiation therapy four to six weeks after the surgery.

The proton-beam facility, on the Harvard University campus, occupied an old, relatively small, single-story, red-brick building, constructed in the 1940s to house the cyclotron. Only a limited number of patients could be treated at any one time, and they were distributed by protocol to different body areas. A new proton-beam machine and setting were being constructed in downtown Boston, but they were not yet operational. Dr. O'Brien reported that there were software problems still being worked out, and the machine would have to be tested for a year or so before patient treatment could begin. All the work currently done in the old facility was research oriented, and I was eligible for treatment through funding provided by the federal government under the guidelines for an experimental protocol.

O'Brien was very thorough in answering all our questions. He seemed to enjoy the process, which permitted him to speak of his research and to express enthusiasm for his work and the different variables he dealt with. I had read his article five or six times and closely inquired into the findings and whatever subsequent data he had collected. It turned out there was a significant difference in the recent effectiveness of the chemotherapy part of the protocol: For unclear reasons, in the past several years, it had been much less effective in shrinking the tumors of my type. But the total sample was too small (eight or nine) for any conclusions to be drawn. After our extended question and answer, O'Brien looked at my films, which included a recent postsurgical MRI. Viewing these scans, he saw a few surprising things. He believed he could affirmatively identify remaining pieces of tumor, at the clivus in particular. He noted that surgeons often believe they have accomplished more than they have, although that hadn't been his prior experience with Dr. Neria. He also indicated that had I been referred to him before my surgery, he would have recommended a course of chemotherapy and radiation to precede surgical intervention. He argued this position from the results of his research, which he assumed Dr. Neria was aware of. Following my surgery, tumor specimens had been tested in the lab against several chemotherapy agents. The assay results, which indicated a probability that I would not be responsive to the conventional chemotherapy cocktail, did not sway O'Brien from his standard protocol.

Treatment by the proton beam would involve my staying in Boston for at least one six-week period; I would also have to come up for preparatory work and some follow-up. The daily routine required two doses of radiation (a combination of photon and proton beams), administered at two different facilities at a considerable distance from one another in the city. O'Brien stated he thought the proton beam was more likely to eliminate the tumor and to be safer. He believed I would be taking a risk with any other treatment.

O'Brien was quite convincing. He was intelligent, articulate, and open. I thus strenuously attempted to relegate my personal convenience, including the anticipated loneliness and disruption of family life, to the background. I was close to being persuaded, and, as we were leaving to go see Dr. Neria, I told Dr. O'Brien we would call in a few days to schedule my treatment. He said he would be away until the following week, as he was visiting Disney World. Having had a one-day experience in that wonderland, I said, with modulated enthusiasm, "Oh, how old are your children?" O'Brien replied that he had none, but his wife had been pressuring him to go. I nodded but could not help but ponder: If you have the opportunity to travel and you don't have kids, why go there? A hint of the incongruous and the absurd entered. Here I was painstakingly evaluating the man, his knowledge and wisdom, and something dissonant intruded from another quarter, for which he indirectly appealed not to be held responsible.

Start Spreading the News

Suzie and I scooted over to the Brigham for our appointment with Neria. On the way, we discussed O'Brien's view of the MRI and the possible arrangements we would make for me to be in Boston for at least six weeks. I had foreseen that our investigating the option of the proton beam would lead to a difficult decision, but this in no way allayed my anxiety.

As Dr. Neria began his physical exam, he asked about our consultations with the radiation oncologists. When I reported O'Brien's perspective on the recent MRI, Neria immediately looked at the films. Disputing O'Brien's conclusions, he asserted that any abnormality that appeared at the clivus was very likely the result of the surgery:

the irregularity in the bone (which was notably at a right angle, the result of resection), the inflammation, and the scar tissue. While it was impossible to determine that there were no cancerous cells or tissue in that location, there was no reason to claim otherwise. Having been there during the surgery and having reviewed the films, Dr. Neria believed that the MRI supported his experience of having removed the entire tumor.

When I described O'Brien's perspective on his treatment protocol, Neria also disagreed. He noted that the present-day "standard of care" (i.e., the consensus of the medical community) for my tumor type was that surgery, if it could be accomplished effectively and safely, should precede the other treatment modalities. He said that O'Brien's treatment was still experimental. He took no position on the relative value of the two radiation methods, although he did say he was not aware of any evidence that the proton beam was more effective with my kind of tumor. He also gave some emphasis to the significance of my relation of trust with Dan. Neria stated he was always available for further consultations and if I ever wanted him to review films. He remarked that one should never trust one radiologist's report or one person's reading.

I consulted with Dan before and after going up to Boston. His view of the MRI was entirely consistent with Neria's. I carefully questioned him regarding the relative merits of the available treatments. I asked him to speak with Dr. O'Brien in order to sharply focus their differences. Dan reported to me that he and O'Brien did differ, but also had much in common. In fact, several years ago, they had simultaneously and separately developed similar ways of safely distributing and controlling radiation in the head.

Dan had formally reviewed the data and a paper that Dr. O'Brien presented at a conference. Dan told me that he himself had successfully treated, with no recurrence, over 20 tumors of my type, which was now described as an esthesioneuroblastoma, there being more elements (though not all) that lined up with such a pathology. He thought there might be a marginal benefit to the proton beam but not one that was scientifically demonstrated or statistically significant.

I decided to be treated with the radiation available in New York. My relationship with Dan and my desire to be followed in my home town played a big part, as did my belief that there was nothing definitive about the superior effectiveness of the proton beam. I was also swayed by the discrepancy in the readings of the MRI and what I felt to be the more consistent and plausible perspective of Neria and Dan. In addition, I felt O'Brien's protocol might be skewing his vision. I was of course influenced by wanting to stay home. I tried to minimize this desire but knew it played a part. I had some misgivings but reconciled myself to them.

Return of the Stuffed Animal

I contacted patients in mid December to inform them of
my plan to return to work in January and then to take another leave for February and March, the duration of the radiation treatment and, following that, a couple weeks for
recovery. The radiation oncologists I had spoken with had
cautioned me not to return to work too soon, and I didn't
want later to postpone my date of return and shift expectations. In mid December, when I made the decision, I was
still recovering from the surgery, with residual feelings of
fatigue and minor but persistent discomfort in my face:
congestion in the nose, excessive tearing in the eyes, numbness in the areas where the incision had been made. The

166

swelling following the surgery continued to decline and my appearance was still changing daily.

I had several qualms about returning for a limited period in January, and I discussed them with colleagues. I wondered whether my temporary return would be useful or productive for the patients, and whether it would be so for me. I thought it might revive feelings of attachment and abandonment and permit almost no time to discuss them. I considered that the several-week resumption of work was significantly motivated by my own desire for contact and connection. I wondered if it had primarily to do with my financial interests (I did not have adequate liability insurance) and my wanting to hold on to my patients.

I worried that my life and concerns would be a primary focus. The preceding period had been very destabilizing: My self-reserve had been punctured in the fall and many aspects of my self-restraint had been subverted. I expected that my present emotional state and physical condition might also be intrusive. Still, I decided that making contact with my patients would be valuable: to inform them of the present circumstances, to demonstrate that I had come through the surgery well, and to convey that resuming our work soon was a probability.

Many of my first returning sessions were very emotional. On initially greeting almost all my patients, I had an urge to hug them, which I suppressed. I gradually realized how fragile and guarded I felt, and how much of my behavior was influenced by a desire to contain my feelings of vulnerability and dependence.

I adopted a general principle of directly responding to patients' inquiries about the status of my illness. While I tried to take their cues in regard to what information they wanted and how much, discerning such cues was difficult, if not impossible. I was intent (perhaps too much so) on allaying their fears of my imminent demise. I wanted to project a reassuring presence and to foster belief in my continuity. But I was not sure what was for my benefit alone and what was for our respective benefits. I was still awash in feelings of exhilaration and anxiety, of intense pleasure in my own survival, and of continuing fear. I felt impulses to hide some aspects of my experience and to share others, and no doubt drew comfort from doing so. But I was equally on guard not to play exclusively into my patients' wish for me to be protected and safe.

This catalogue of emotions included a high degree of instability and uncertainty. It was accompanied by an assumption that in this short period nothing could be reconciled, resolved, or adequately uncovered. Because our meetings in January constituted only a temporary reunion, I anticipated that patients would probably still be inhibiting their distress and anger at my unavailability. I was aware they would feel preempted and powerless, manipulated and quite vulnerable in their attachment. The peculiar parameters of the therapeutic relationship, the boundaries that protected my private life, were palpable and frustrating to many of them.

These feelings were reflected in my work with Ellen, the 27-year-old woman who had given me her stuffed dog. When I greeted her in the waiting room at our first session in January, I wanted to hug her. I registered the impulse but reacted by presenting a reserved demeanor. In the past Ellen had at times expressed a desire for us to hug and dismay that I wouldn't oblige her. She had spoken openly of romantic and erotic feelings for me, but had also acknowledged that the prospect of such feelings being mutual would make her feel unsafe. She had for a while, in order to protect herself, secretly maintained some uncertainty as to my sexual orientation. She bridled at her awareness that I was married and blamed the therapeutic situation (and me) for stirring feelings within her that could not be resolved. She often worried over her place in my life; she wanted to be first and foremost, desired above all, only to feel dissatisfied, disappointed, and hurt on realizing that she wasn't.

All this contributed to my internal struggle around my feelings of attraction to Ellen and concerns that I was being seductive, that I induced feelings of affection and attachment that were jumbled up with erotic longings as well. These complications were being sorted out, although many had not been explicitly recognized and acknowledged. I had been wary of physical contact, was guarded, and had maintained a clear boundary. In this moment, however, I had a powerful urge to embrace her, an urge that I identified as clearly emerging from within myself.

Ellen's father adored her as a young child, but he also was limited and tantalizing in his attentions. He left her mother and Ellen for another woman when Ellen was seven, and he was, thereafter, very harmfully inconsistent in his capacity to be present: He solicited Ellen's attachment and adoration only to abandon her repeatedly. She would make plans with him, then wonder why he didn't show up; he would offer a pathetic and implausible litany of excuses. She also felt guilty for her inclination to abandon *him*. Her confounding experience of his untrustworthiness had resulted in an endless cycle of yearning for priority and attention, only to reexperience abandonment and rejection.

Ellen had been distraught at my illness and, on my return, I felt some responsibility, even guilt, for the fear and anguish that my crisis and departure had elicited. I had been utterly unavailable and preoccupied with my own survival and held her at a considerable distance, if at all.

At the outset of our first January session, I returned the stuffed dog. I was not comfortable with its presence in a drawer in my office; I was not using it or caring for it; I did not consciously want to hold it or to hold on to it. I felt duplicitous keeping it. I had accepted the dog with a mixture of gratitude and reluctance, and I handed it back to Ellen with like emotions. She felt I did so abruptly and coldly. When she expressed her unhappiness with my manner of returning it, I acknowledged I had felt burdened by its presence. I had been unsure whether I could give it back, let alone care for it. I had felt that it offered me no comfort, that her gesture involved a denial of the circumstances of my life and illness, a wish for magical protection that left me more isolated than connected. I could not hold her or it. I recognized a callousness in my response, an inability to appreciate and accept her gesture, something of a dismissal of the feeling of an embrace, of a symbol of being held. I had been unable to leave behind my limited and anxious perspective.

Ellen and I have discussed these feelings many times. She has chided me about my reserve and restraint, and I have expressed regret about how I handled her stuffed animal. Ellen has reminded me that shortly before my illness she had a dream in which she went back to her father's house (in which he lived with his new wife and child and stepchildren) and retrieved her stuffed dog. She had seen the dream, particularly the recovery of her animal, as a tangible representation of the work we were doing together. She had taken pains in deciding what to give me at the time of my medical leave and chose "doggie" as the most personal expression possible of her love and gratitude. Ellen remembered that when she handed me the stuffed animal she said, "If it wasn't for you, I wouldn't have been able to get it back." She saw her gesture as sustaining the possibility of my taking care of her and of her taking care of me, even in my absence.

There have been many times when I have wanted the dog back in order to hold it differently. Sometimes I think I am the dog.

In Human Hands

The radiation was no walk in the woods, despite the fact that about 30 square feet of wallpaper on the ceiling of the radiation room depicted the intertwining branches of several trees. From where I lay when I was being zapped, I looked up through the plastic mesh of a tight-fitting mask that was clamped to the table. The continuity of the wallpaper and of the budding branches was punctuated by more than one electrical outlet and device. I traveled by subway to and from this room, which, situated in the hospital's basement, was separated only by some walls from one of the city's largest subway interchanges (Union Square). The radiation room itself reminded me of a medieval castle's torture chamber, lined with shelves carrying the carefully molded personal appurtenances to hold each patient in the proper posture of submission, along with the personally molded lead blocks designed to direct the individual destructive rays.

My comrades, almost all women with breast cancer and men with prostate cancer, sat in a small area waiting to be called for their daily dose. A bemused and mordant air tended to reign. I endured all the expected side effects, but worse was the extended inactivity and blanket fatigue. I became noticeably depressed for a period of time. I was exhausted, worn down, and cut off and considered myself utterly inessential and dispensable.

During the course of the radiation treatment, the volume of the now-excised tumor was carefully evaluated to see whether or not additional radiation using different technology (stereotactic surgery) made sense. This involved still more exacting filming of my brain and skull. Dan informed me that in his assessment and that of his colleagues, the stereotactic surgery would not be necessary. This was a matter of "physics," of calculations done by computer. Dan said, and I believed him, that the mathematics were too complicated to convey and too difficult for me to understand. As prior to the outset of the radiation Dan had thought this additional radiation would likely be called for, I was somewhat uneasy. I tried to grasp the nonmathematical logic of the decision making but came to accept that, beyond the most general description of the variables of dose, tolerance, angles and volumes, I could not know or understand the details. I trusted Dan.

At the completion of the radiation I met with him for our weekly checkup. After assuring me that I had received the maximum dose of radiation that the different areas could tolerate, Dan said, "I don't know what your beliefs are, but at this point many patients find it comforting or helpful to think that now they are in God's hands." I didn't: "That's not the way I think of it. I've been glad to be in human hands . . . that human hands were available to me. . . . I've been glad to be in your hands."

Life Without Parole

When I returned to work in early April, it felt like a reprieve. But how I would be let out of confinement was partially up to the parole board of my patients, and almost all of them wanted initially to diminish the frequency of their sessions. Their reasoning was virtually unanimous. It was very hard to make the transition to working together again. They didn't trust in my presence and continuity. They had all lived with the prospect of my death, of coping with the anticipated loss, of distracting themselves from it.

At our first session following my leave, Ben, the fiction writer who was terrified and appeared distant at our parting, presented me with a chapter of a novel he had begun, a chapter in a first-person narrative with a focus on the protagonist's imagined conversations with his dead therapist, David. These conversations are alternately open, anxious, and playful regarding the intimacy and influence of the relationship. They are passionate, humorous, angry, and tender, and they are described as almost endless. In fact, their endlessness is a problem for the central character, analogous to his sleeplessness. He strives to make the dialogues go on and on, while also attempting to be realistic and thus face an imaginary therapy session's arbitrary ending. The ongoing internal dialogues present the participants as being in a struggle of wills and vulnerabilities. The narrator describes a tense identification with his therapist, particularly in the questions he asks himself and in the therapist's responses which he invents. He describes feelings of anger, hostility, and aggressiveness toward the therapist, irritation at the latter's power and smugness, but also sharp feelings of guilt.

As I read the chapter, I was deeply moved and took pleasure in the depiction of the vital bond between the patient and therapist, in and outside each other's presence. I saw that a form of survival for the dead therapist was at stake and that Ben was profoundly involved in sensing and reflecting on the many qualities of our relationship. I was comforted by his decidedly forthright acknowledgment of our connection and its importance (which had seemed lacking at the time of my departure). His gesture in handing me the chapter was generous, as was the openness of its contents.

When we spoke later, looking backward with the benefit of time, Ben reported that, on my return, he was most struck by the changes in my appearance. He remembered me as being gaunt, seeming to be physically fragile, breakable. Acknowledging that he felt very awkward about having killed me off in his novel, he spoke about the paradoxical nature of the boundaries in our relationship: how he felt them to be very protective, providing him with safety and security and the assurance that he would be listened to, that he could speak freely about things, that the distinct beginning and ending of sessions were like the confines of a poem. But he also felt that the boundaries were strictly enforced by me in a way that had limited his responsiveness to me, that they had contributed to his coldness and detachment in the autumn of my illness. He felt that the shape of the relationship, the hierarchy, the way power was distributed, had inherently qualified his ability to respond sympathetically and emotionally to me. He also acknowledged his tendency to be self-protective, that often his feelings unfolded and gained expression only slowly over time. When my illness intervened, we had no such time.

Another patient, Greg, told me that my illness and description of my pursuit of medical opinions had led him to attend to some relatively minor physical ailments of his own. What followed was the traumatic uncovering of a form of leukemia and then his arranging for immediate treatment. In my absence he had undergone a course of chemotherapy that was effective, and he had a good prognosis. Greg's former retreat before doctors and his difficulties coping with the prospect of ongoing care had been affected by our discussions of my situation.

My patient Roland and I spoke further about the significant role he had played in my finding Dr. Neria. I expressed my deep gratitude. Roland's manner, in this instance, was to minimize the significance of his gesture and his considerable help. One aspect of our exchanges in the past had been my questioning the ways he extended himself for others, particularly as he often complained he was taken for granted. I believe I had previously taken some of his caring and attentiveness for granted as well. His extraordinary aid in regard to my illness brought to prominence this poorly recognized side of his self.

As a child Roland had been physically abused by his father and, in effect, abandoned by his mother, who herself was under considerable duress because of his father. At the time of my illness, his response was to be quiet and reserved, except for his singular act of generosity.

Several other patients were quite angry at what they experienced as having been put on hold. Patients who had been designated caretakers within their families resented being encumbered with concern for my well-being. Others felt cast adrift and displaced. Yet there was a striking persistence in the face of the difficulties. Our intimate connection had survived a profound disruption, one that emphasized the patients' being on the outside of my life, deprived of the ordinary means of contact between people. Many disparities in our relative positions had been laid bare. Several patients commented that my illness and absence had disrupted certain illusions they had persistently held on to, particularly their sense of priority in my consciousness and in my life.

There thus was a caution and tentativeness surrounding the resumption of work. There were questions regarding my physical stamina, and a bit of testing, sometimes overtly playful, to see if my memory and mind had been impaired. My appearance was significantly different. I shaved the beard I had maintained for 25 years, as the radiation had permanently eliminated my mustache. There was a large swatch of hair missing from the back of my head, a temporary result of the radiation (its exit point). I had an impulse to hide the back of my head, and my following my patients from the waiting room to my office now had a new motivation. I wanted to obscure the effects of the treatment and of my vulnerability.

By July, three months later, all the patients had resumed coming at their earlier frequency. However, in the middle of the month I unexpectedly had to have my right tear duct reconstructed. I had had recurrent swelling and infections. The relatively minor surgery was not planned, so I was unable to give my patients notice prior to my two-day absence. For one patient this separation was unbearable, and she ended her work with me. She had an older sister who had died in her 40s from a brain tumor, and her mother was chronically physically and mentally ill. This patient, who had begun work with me only a few weeks before I took my medical leave in October, had decided to wait for my return, despite being offered referrals. She had found two covering therapists woefully deficient. Her anger at me reached a crescendo around the canceled session in July. She felt that I had been curt and cavalier in my phone call to her (made from the hospital), that I had failed to provide her with an adequate and acceptable reason for my absence and to offer her an alternative appointment time. Our joint efforts to acknowledge each other's circumstances and to make reparation were unsuccessful.

Another patient, prompted by the canceled session in July, also announced her intention to find another therapist. She too felt I had been inattentive and callous, and she could no longer tolerate dealing with my illness. She described how seeing me impaired her ability to focus on herself and seemed to diminish and silence her concerns. She was increasingly doubtful that she could resolve with me her longstanding fears of being abandoned. She thought I might not be operating at full capacity, and this possibility was too intrusive and disruptive for her. She decided to continue for a while, although aware that her guilt at separating significantly contributed to the decision.

The July reconstruction of my tear duct served to illuminate a third patient's experience of what might be referred to as his deathwatch. Tom, described earlier as a patient particularly attuned to my more internal emotional states, was the one who, not yet informed of my illness, had complained, "Something is wrong with you!" As we spoke about my recent minor surgery in July, it became apparent that he remained quite confused about my general status and prognosis. Although I had been intent on being straightforward and clear in January and April, Tom had somehow continued to assume that my survival was questionable on an almost moment-by-moment basis. I was surprised that he had been speaking to me in that context. As an adolescent Tom had endured the ordeal of two elder siblings becoming schizophrenic, and he was used to living in a hazy atmosphere of the unacknowledged and the precarious.

When we later discussed what had gone on between us, Tom was reminded that at the time his sister had her first psychotic break and was hospitalized, he had no idea; it was as though she just disappeared. When she returned home and stayed in her room, no one told him what had happened; no one said anything. In the fall, when I told him of my illness, he at first wondered, "Should I know this?" and initially felt that he would have preferred being left in the dark. Following my "disappearance," he felt implicated and guilty and carried around with him the stark sensation that he had caused it. After my return he continued to feel as if we were hanging on the edge of a cliff. Only retrospectively did he recognize the extent of his bitterness, hostility, and anger, but also his despair about having a damaged capacity to know distinctly enough what he experienced.

Tom had sensed something was amiss when it was not yet explicit and then, later, didn't know or couldn't accept the reported success of my treatment when I had sought to impress it upon him. There, too, he had likely picked up on a subterranean stream of my continuing uncertainty and anxiety.

False Bottom

*O*ne year after learning of my tumor, 10 months after the surgery, and six months after the completion of the radiation, I went with Suzie to an appointment with Dan, my radiation oncologist. I had had an MRI of my brain and sinus cavities the preceding week. It was at an interval of four months from my previous MRI. The earlier scan was something of a baseline: The radiation, like the surgery, had created scar tissue and mucus, thus making the reading of the films difficult. Dan had reported to me in May that, as far as they could tell, there was no indication of tumor. He had said that we could wait six months before repeating the scan, but if I wanted we could do it sooner.

So, on September 11th, Suzie and I were ushered into a consulting room about 45 minutes after our appointment time. My chart was placed in a transparent holder on the room door, with the radiologist's report attached to its front with a paper clip. Suzie and I both immediately read the report, which contained the following sentences: "There has been *interval increase* in the volume of the mildly enhancing, abnormal soft tissue *most consistent with tumor,* which replaces the clivus and extends into the prepontine cistern posteriorly and into the left parapharyngeal space anterolaterally." Given the proximity of the clivus to the brain stem, tumor progression meant I was in considerable danger.

Suzie and I read and reread those lines a half-dozen times in the 45 more minutes we waited before Dan's appearance. I paced back and forth, periodically cursing, entering into the feeling state of the previous autumn. While I was thinking about options and possible actions, I was also imagining that I might soon be faced with symptoms and severe illness, and, relatively soon, with death. A nurse entered the room and asked me several questions, and when I mentioned the report and my terror, he seemed not to hear what I said.

At last Dan entered the office and cheerily asked, "How are you?" I told him that we had read the radiologist's report, to which he simply stated that he hadn't. He picked it up and looked at it. He then proceeded to compound his oversight: "If this is so, we'll have to see what options are available.... You know ... last fall I didn't think surgery was possible, so if there is progression of the tumor I think that surgery would be highly unlikely.... You've received about as much radiation as the area can tolerate, so I don't think we can do much in that respect. There is, of course, chemo-therapy which ... well ... we have to see. I think we should send the films up to Dr. Neria and I will look at them. .... I will call you tomorrow." He repeated variants of these statements a few times and assured me I would hear from him.

Suzie and I lived the next day in despair and terror. I re-played all the decisions I had made regarding my treatments and subjected them to renewed scrutiny. I anticipated with utter dread another round of consultations. I was thrown outside all my assumptions and reeled in disbelief. That af-ternoon and evening I saw several patients and once again felt I was bluffing. While I knew enough not to give credi-bility to just one doctor's reading of the films (and recalled Dr. Neria's warning), I lived nonetheless with the possibil-ity that this first opinion was accurate. I again imagined dis-appearing from my children's lives. I felt isolated and assaulted and was unable to sleep.

Dan called me late in the morning of the next day and began by saying, "I'm probably the only person who got less sleep than you did last night" (which would not have been possible). He said that he had looked at the scans with the neuroradiologist he ordinarily works with, and they concurred that there had been no change since my last MRI. The first report had been written by a less experi-enced and less discriminating radiologist. Despite my con-siderable experience, I was still surprised at how much doctors could differ in what they saw. Dan asked a few times if there was anything he could do to provide me with more assurance. I asked that we meet, as I wanted him to look at the films with us. Dan answered, "David, you can't read the films!" I acknowledged this reality, but added that I wanted to hear him tell me what he saw, to hear what he had to say in person. Dan acceded to my request, and we made an appointment for the early morning two days later.

At that time, Dan took Suzie and me to meet Dr. Lucene, the more experienced neuroradiologist who had been away the preceding week owing to the death of her father. As we walked down the hospital corridors and chatted, Dan continued to be quite defensive about what had happened earlier that week. Suzie suggested that perhaps in the future an unread radiologist's report not be left out for patients to read. Apparently missing the implications of her remark, Dan argued that he wanted his patients to be well informed and saw no harm in that. He also defensively asserted that leaving the charts out was something he was proud of because it facilitated the smooth running of the office. While professing to understand how terrified we were, he never simply apologized.

Dr. Lucene had my MRIs up on two computers. She showed that there was no significant difference in the sets from May and September. She identified where she thought the other radiologist had mistakenly read changes and had misidentified locations. She graciously solicited all our questions. Just before we left her office, Dan leaned over and, pointing out how close the tumor had been to the brain stem, noted the scale of the picture and what appeared to be one or two millimeters distance. One week later, Dr. Neria concurred with the more encouraging view of the recent scans.

This experience shook me up and put me in a place I had come to detest. A latent anxiety, some of which I was not conscious of, surged to the surface. Once again I was shocked at the location of the tumor. I was angry at how dependent I was on a doctor who seemed so overworked and inattentive.

Referring to Dan's neglect, my friend Eric remarked that I didn't deserve this, which elicited from me, "I don't know that I want to live in a world where people get what they deserve." Eric also jokingly wondered whether I was familiar with an essay by a Kleinian psychoanalyst regarding addiction to near-death experience.

Coming and Going Before the Graveyard

Another two months later and 11 days following a new MRI, I had my next scheduled consultation with Dan. He met with us accompanied by two visiting radiation oncologists and two nurse practitioners. He chattered about the presidential election and the validity of his patient polls and prattled on about the Yankees. After completion of my physical exam, Dan said he thought we should schedule a new MRI. In disbelief, I told him that I had just had one and, fortunately, had already received a call from Dr. Lucene that this set of scans continued to exhibit no change. Dan acknowledged that he had neither read the report nor viewed the films. He was vague about exactly when he had been away on a trip and told me he would call the following day. I was stupefied and said little.

As we left the office, I recognized the intensity of my anger. In the moment, in his office, I felt trapped and had been almost paralyzed. When I didn't hear from Dan the next day, I called him. I told him that I was disturbed and upset about what had happened the previous day. Dan and I then went around in circles several times. I stated that it was my understanding that the consultation had been set up in relation to my getting the MRI, that it was my expectation that he read the films, that it was very important to me that he do so soon after they were taken, and that he give a carefully considered opinion. Dan answered by telling me how overwhelmed with work he was, that he had been traveling for business the preceding week, that he had 300 to 400 patients he was following, that on the given Monday when he returned to his office he had some 50 films to look at. He said he had not looked at my chart before meeting with me and thus didn't know I had had the scan and, in any event, couldn't be expected to know when a particular patient was having a scan done. I repeated what my expectation was, particularly following my experience in September. Again Dan did not simply say, "I'm sorry," which would have satisfied me. Rather, he offered, "If you want me to apologize, I'll apologize." But he added that he couldn't promise it wouldn't happen again. He was well aware of the extent of his responsibilities, he continued, he took them on willingly, and I should know by now that he fulfilled them, that he did his job. I told him that I was very grateful for the wonderful things he had done for me in the past, how he had extended himself in very significant ways, all of which meant a great deal to me. But I also conveyed that I was depending on him to follow me closely, that he was the primary doctor looking after me now, something about which he had seemed uncertain. Dan claimed he was aware of this. He didn't rush to get off the phone but lingered well after I thought we had presented our perspectives.

Over the course of the preceding year, Dan had been at times atypically and remarkably available and accessible—and when I needed him most. On several later occasions he had been present in a more perfunctory fashion, when I was assumed to be in a safer place. In our last meeting it seemed as though he had little idea who I was (i.e., the patient who two months earlier had been terrified by an unread radiologist's report). Of course his distance may reflect the impossible workload he had taken on. As there was now no apparent urgency in my case, with everything assumed to be okay, I was consigned to the background of his consciousness.

Following my phone conversation with Dan, I reflected on the fact that he had tried to count on my deference and his authority to argue that my minimal expectations of clinical engagement were excessive: He defended a kind of clinical practice that I assumed he would never teach his students. Rather than being diverted by Yankee and election chatter, I would have much preferred that he had taken 30 seconds to review my chart before meeting with me and then taken an additional two or three minutes to read the radiologist's report. The pretense of personal contact I can do without.

Life-and-Death Dialogues

*I*n my talking with doctors I was not looking for Shangri-la. Nor was I just like Pooh tracking a woozle. In those life-and-death dialogues, I was looking for a way of ascertaining real tracks, of finding out what could be reasonably discerned. I was seeking to identify the contours of what I was faced with. In my case, part of the reality of what I sought, that which existed outside and independent of me, also lay inside my head. It had grown to take up the empty spaces in my skull.

Five years have elapsed since the surgery and there has been no recurrence of the cancer, although there has been plenty of recurrence, in my mind, of the talking I did with doctors.

Absurd as it may have been—although inevitable once thrust into the situation—I spoke with and evaluated most of the doctors in the context of a highly pressured and time-limited single interaction. In these conversations there was no safe haven, no illusory security, and I used every means available to me—perceptual, affective, cognitive— to gauge the physician. I tried to assess his or her prepara- tion, calm, and observational acuity, his or her degree of confidence, control, and purposiveness. I was attentive to professional and personal discipline and to the capacity for self-reflection. I wanted someone who paid meticulous at- tention to detail and was comprehensive, someone who was neither distracted nor too adamant. I preferred a doc- tor who was willing to communicate his or her reasoning, who wanted to explain and was able to do so. I wanted a doctor who was responsive and took me and my questions seriously; I was looking for someone who was collaborative both with his or her fellow physicians and with me.

I tended, at times, to focus on issues of logic and lan- guage, but by no means exclusively. I assessed the individual physician's reasoning, three-dimensional problem solving, and the ways in which these were articulated; I also took in the doctor's voice and physical presence and gestures. I felt that who a doctor was as a person could be very relevant to his or her action and behavior as a physician; I tried to sense who the individual was.

These assembled "criteria," unformulated at the time, constitute something of a retrospective wish list, not one that I ever organized or expected to be entirely fulfilled. I may have been looking for the physician who had the great- est capacity to perceive and differentiate in my case, plus all the other desirable attributes, yet I also qualified and contained the wish in several ways. I reminded myself that individuals are variously skilled and there can be considerable inconsistency in the degree to which they excel at distinct tasks. In other words, a doctor could be a master in the operating room and quite quirky outside it. I reflected on some of Proust's characters: most gifted in one realm, least so in others. I thought about how the total personality of the doctor did not necessarily matter, was not necessarily involved. I acknowledged my own fallibility, as well as that of the physicians. I considered that many of the desirable attributes were *not* requirements.

My primary-care doctor had remarked, upon his entrance onto the scene, that my medical predicament was "over [his] head." Several of the other physicians whom I spoke with personally, who were not oncology specialists, commented similarly. I took this to mean that my specific illness was well beyond their area of expertise and that they were cautious and uncertain about how much direction they could provide. Yet I felt it was therefore all the more vital that I have several such doctors to talk with. These nononcology physicians served the distinct purpose of supporting my layman's position. I used our conversations and their general medical knowledge to bolster myself as someone with a relatively solid basis for inquiry. Also, being physicians, they readily accepted that doctors have conflicts and failings; not being oncology specialists, they were not in competition with any of the other physicians. Along with my nonmedical colleagues, they collectively helped to provide me with greater freedom of thought and movement. I therefore became an avid solicitor of help.

The path to a decision regarding treatment lay through the many thickets of patient–physician conversations, dialogues that have few rivals for density, opaqueness, and uncertainty. To find a viable remedy (and the best physician) involved pushing through all sorts of thorny areas—my feelings of dependence, ignorance, powerlessness, and despair *and* the doctors' defensiveness, pretense of disinterest, and occasional misuse of power and authority. There were also the thickets of films and their interpretations, of readings and misreadings, and the physicians' variability of perception.

Of course I could not evaluate in a fully empirical or objective fashion. Of course any method of inquiry or means of perception would also be defensive and self-preservative. Of course, in any dialogue, each person can have very different impressions of what has occurred (even one person can, at the same or different times). Certainly, some things I could never know.

But in the consultation process, the trials and tribulations of interpretation by the doctors and of the doctors ultimately had to come to an end. While there necessarily was some leeway in comprehending images on an MRI or CT scan, I had to decide which interpretations seemed more right than others. Whatever awareness I had that my perspectives and experience were relative and constructed did not contradict the desire to see and to know for myself.

To let a physician inside my skull to within a millimeter of my brain stem, to put my life so thoroughly in someone else's hands, I wanted to trust the person, and I wanted to trust my own judgment. This desire persisted despite my relative ignorance and the continuous feeling that I was "flying blind," that a wild storm was raging and I did not know the coordinates of my position or my destination.

I was fortunate to have gained considerable experience reviewing dialogues and interactions, identifying lapses and inconsistencies and maneuvers that guided and misguided interpersonal exchanges. It helped that I was aware that a doctor's self-interest and character can facilitate or interfere with a patient's treatment. I recognized, too, that I had to go against the grain of many of my impulses, particularly those to turn away, relent, and avoid confrontation.

Looking back, I realize that I scrutinized, replayed, and reconsidered much of my interaction with the doctors in a fashion that corresponded with how I attended to sessions with patients. Doing so was a means of protection, of countering my feelings of powerlessness, as well as a manner of engaging with experience, of working and playing with what I heard and saw and felt. This correspondence, I now see, was in the process of talking with doctors: the inquiry, the waiting, the tolerance for anxiety, the hope of discovery—a process that made it possible for me to sort out what could be known. With the aid of other people, my abilities to discern and decide were not fatally compromised.

I appreciate the distinctive circumstances of my individual case. I was fortunate in the timely discovery of the tumor and about its particular pathology. I was lucky that I wasn't experiencing debilitating symptoms that would have prevented extensive consultation. It was my good luck that I had the amount of time that I did, along with adequate medical insurance which paid for more than 95% of my treatment. Cost-containment strictures and inequities in the availability of care were not harmful in my case, as they are in so many others. I had a wife and family and friends and colleagues who were helpful and on whom I could rely;

I had friends who were doctors with whom I could regularly speak. Together they helped me to overcome many of the impersonal factors in contemporary medical care. For those with less adequate resources and fewer or even no people to turn to, there is too often no means of protection from impersonal treatment provided by detached, authoritative, and inaccessible individuals.

It worked to my advantage that there was delay and confusion and pretense on Mount Olympus (which, I now recall, was quite typical of the Greek deities). My own patient's referral to Dr. Neria was fortuitous as well—no doctor with whom I directly consulted referred me to the person I found to be the best physician.

I needed help, I sought help, and, remarkably, I found it. I am alive, as are all three of my children, because of the intervention of doctors. I am immensely grateful I have been in human hands.

Notes

[1]To cite a few significant and representative papers:

Aron, Lewis (1991), The patient's experience of the analyst's subjectivity. *Psychoanal. Dial.,* 1:29–51.

Benjamin, Jessica (1990), Recognition and destruction: An outline of intersubjectivity. *Psychoanal. Psychol.,* 7(Suppl.):33–47.

Hoffman, Irwin Z. (1983), The patient as interpreter of the analyst's experience. *Contemp. Psychoanal.,* 19:389–422.

Ogden, Thomas (1994), The analytic third: Working with intersubjective clinical facts. *Internat. J. Psycho-Anal.,* 75:3–19.

Renik, Owen (1993), Analytic interaction: Conceptualizing technique in light of the analyst's irreducible subjectivity. *Psychoanal. Quart.,* 62:553–571.

All these essays can be found in:

Mitchell, Stephen A. & Aron, Lewis, eds. (1999), *Relational Psychoanalysis: The Emergence of a Tradition*. Hillsdale, NJ: The Analytic Press.

[2]Prior to my illness I had not read any articles regarding serious illness in the therapist, but I was familiar with an edited collection of essays that dealt with how crises in a therapist's private life affected his or her work:

Gerson, Barbara, ed. (1996), *The Analyst as a Person*. Hillsdale, NJ: The Analytic Press.

After my surgery, another collection was brought to my attention:

Schwartz, H. J. & Silver, A.-L. S., eds. (1990), *Illness in the Analyst: Implications for the Treatment Relationship*. New York: International Universities Press.

There is also now a growing literature on the interaction between patient and therapist when the latter is seriously ill or dying. The articles I have found most helpful and thought- provoking are:

Fajardo, Barbara (2001), Life-threatening illness in the analyst. *J. Amer. Psychoanal. Assn.,* 49:569–586.
Feinsilver, J. L. (1997), The therapist as a person facing death: The hardest of external realities and therapeutic action. *Internat. J. Psycho-Anal.,* 79:1131–1150.
Hoffman, Irwin Z. (2000), At death's door: Therapists and patients as agents. *Psychoanal. Dial.,* 10:823–846.
Morrison, Amy Lichtblau (1997), Ten years of doing psychotherapy while living with a life-threatening illness: Self-disclosure and other ramifications. *Psychoanal. Dial.,* 7:215–240.
Pizer, Barbara (1997), When the analyst is ill: Dimensions of self-disclosure. *Psychoanal. Quart.,* 66:450–469.

Acknowledgments

There are many people who helped me through the course of my illness and many who have helped in the evolution of this book.

I would like to acknowledge the graciousness, generosity, and editorial acumen of Paul Stepansky, Managing Director of The Analytic Press. From the outset of our contact, Paul has conveyed warmth and kindness, along with keen intelligence and intense involvement. I, and the manuscript, have benefited from his wonderful attention.

I want to thank Lew Aron for his essential support and encouragement. I also want to express my gratitude to Liz McNamara, who was immensely helpful with legal advice.

I would like also to thank the following people, some for being there during my illness (and after), some for reading earlier versions of the text, and some for hazarding both: Harriet Barash, Ken Barash, Sue Erikson Bloland, Nina Brodsky, Mel Bukiet, Lorraine Caputo, Ina Cholst, Willa Cobert, Joel Copperman, Mark Danner, Anne de Armas, Donna Demetri-Friedman, Randi Epstein, Elizabeth Fagan, Claudia Fine, Peter Freundlich, Ira Goldberg, Jill Goodman, Sandra Green, Evy Hartman, Geoffrey Hartman, Irwin Hirsch, David Hurwitz, George Igel, Ronnie Igel, Allison Kalfus, Mary Beth Kelly, Jay Kwawer, Lisa Lipman, Liz Marks, Diane Meier, Eric Mendelsohn, Aaron Metrikin, Megan Metrikin, Elisa Owen, Guy Owen, Steven Pollan, Georgette Pan, Barrie Raik, Jerry Raik, Ken Roth, Chris Rothko, Mary Lou Teel, Jim Traub, Mary Jane Waters-Sales, Jessica Weiss, and Debra Worth. I have tried to convey in the manuscript some of the extraordinary help I received.

I would like to thank my patients for their understanding, perseverance, and trust.

I also wish to express my great appreciation and gratitude to the doctors who saved my life.

My thanks to Suzie's mother, Ruth Weiss, and Suzie's brother Joe for their help and presence.

My parents, Robert and Marianne Newman, have always stood by me, deeply connected, loving, and encouraging. I have often turned to my sister Leslie, relied on her, and shared my experience with her.

To Jacob, Isaiah, and Judah, and to Suzie, I dedicate this book.